Individualized In-Vitro Fertilization

T0201408

Individualized In-Vitro Fertilization

Delivering Precision Fertility Treatment

Edited by

Human M. Fatemi
ART Fertility Clinic

Barbara Lawrenz
ART Fertility Clinic

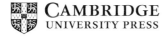

CAMBRIDGE
UNIVERSITY PRESS

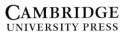

University Printing House, Cambridge CB2 8BS, United Kingdom

One Liberty Plaza, 20th Floor, New York, NY 10006, USA

477 Williamstown Road, Port Melbourne, VIC 3207, Australia

314–321, 3rd Floor, Plot 3, Splendor Forum, Jasola District Centre,
New Delhi – 110025, India

79 Anson Road, #06–04/06, Singapore 079906

Cambridge University Press is part of the University of Cambridge.

It furthers the University's mission by disseminating knowledge in the pursuit of
education, learning, and research at the highest international levels of excellence.

www.cambridge.org
Information on this title: www.cambridge.org/9781108799683
DOI: 10.1017/9781108891622

First published 2021

Printed in the United Kingdom by TJ Books Limited, Padstow Cornwall

A catalogue record for this publication is available from the British Library.

Library of Congress Cataloging-in-Publication Data
Names: Fatemi, Human M., editor. | Lawrenz, Barbara, editor.
Title: Individualized in-vitro fertilization : delivering precision fertility treatment / edited by Human M.
Fatemi, Barbara Lawrenz.
Description: Cambridge, United Kingdom ; New York, NY : Cambridge University Press, 2021. | Includes
bibliographical references and index.
Identifiers: LCCN 2020029466 (print) | LCCN 2020029467 (ebook) | ISBN 9781108799683 (paperback) |
ISBN 9781108891622 (ebook)
Subjects: MESH: Fertilization in Vitro – methods | Precision Medicine – methods | Infertility – therapy
Classification: LCC RG135 (print) | LCC RG135 (ebook) | NLM WQ 208 | DDC 618.1/780599–dc23
LC record available at https://lccn.loc.gov/2020029466
LC ebook record available at https://lccn.loc.gov/2020029467

ISBN 978-1-108-79968-3 Paperback

Contents

Contributors

Diana Alecsandru, MD, PhD, Department of Immunology, IVI RMA Madrid, Spain

Lucía Alegre, MSc, IVF Laboratory, IVI RMA, Valencia, Spain

Samer Alfarawati, Juno Genetics/IVI RMA Global, Oxford, UK

David H. Barad, MD, Center for Human Reproduction, New York, USA; Foundation for Reproductive Medicine, New York, USA

Lorena Bori, MSc, PhD student, IVF Laboratory, IVI RMA, Valencia, Spain

Gustavo Nardini Cecchino, MD, Department of Reproductive Endocrinology and Infertility, IVI RMA Madrid, Spain

Carol Coughlan, MD, ART Fertility Clinics, Dubai, UAE

Neelke De Munck, PhD, MSc, ART Fertility Clinics, Abu Dhabi, UAE

Ibrahim Elkhatib, MSc, ART Fertility Clinics, Abu Dhabi, UAE

Elpida Fragouli, BSc, MSc, PhD, FRSB, FIBMS, Juno Genetics/IVI RMA Global, Oxford, UK; Nuffield Department of Women's and Reproductive Health, University of Oxford, UK

Juan Antonio García Velasco, MD, PhD, Department of Reproductive

Endocrinology and Infertility, IVI RMA Madrid, Spain

Norbert Gleicher, MD, Center for Human Reproduction, New York, USA; Foundation for Reproductive Medicine, New York, USA; Stem Cell Biology and Molecular Embryology Laboratory, Rockefeller University, New York, USA; Department of Obstetrics and Gynecology, Medical University of Vienna, Austria

Irene Hervás, MSc, PhD student, IVF Laboratory, IVI RMA, Valencia, Spain

Luisa Loiudice, MD, IVI RMA, Rome, Italy

Anna Mantzouratou, BSc, MSc, PhD, Life and Environmental Sciences Department, Bournemouth University, UK

Laura Melado, MD, PhD, ART Fertility Clinics, Abu Dhabi, UAE

Marcos Meseguer, MSc, PhD, IVF Laboratory, IVI RMA, Valencia, Spain

Antonio Pellicer, MD, PhD, IVI RMA, Rome, Italy

Matheus Roque, MD, PhD, Mater Prime, Reproductive Medicine, São Paulo, Brazil

Diego Ventura Tarasconi, MD, Department of Reproductive Endocrinology and Infertility, IVI RMA Madrid, Spain

Individualized Ovarian Stimulation for Normal and High Responders

Laura Melado and Human M. Fatemi

1.1 Introduction

Despite the notion that the first baby, Louise Brown, was born in 1978 following IVF performed in a natural menstrual cycle, ovarian stimulation became the gold standard of care in clinical IVF, since the number of oocytes retrieved is directly associated with pregnancy and life birth rates (1, 2). The aim should be to titrate the stimulation in such a way that the optimal number of follicles develops. Too few follicles (also referred to as low response) usually means poor IVF outcome, whereas too many developing follicles induce a risk for developing OHSS and possibly reduce the chance of success with increasing number of oocytes, if stimulation is not adjusted toward the end of the follicular phase (3, 4).

To perform a correct individualization of treatment protocols in IVF, an accurate prediction of ovarian response should be performed, based on the most sensitive markers of ovarian reserve. In this chapter, we discuss the use of the ovarian reserve markers to categorize women based on their anticipated ovarian response. As well, we describe the therapeutic approach and adjustments for an individualized ovarian stimulation for normo- and high responders.

1.2 Evaluation of Ovarian Response

1.2.1 Markers of Ovarian Function

The first step to performing an individualized ovarian stimulation is to evaluate the ovarian response. Accurate and reliable predictors of ovarian reserve are needed to identify patients likely to have poor response, normal response, or hyperresponse to treatment and to guide physicians in selecting the optimal dose of gonadotrophins for ovarian stimulation. To predict ovarian reserve and reproductive potential, several different measures of ovarian reserve have been identified over time, including biochemical measures and ovarian imaging, with varying degrees of success.

Nowadays, the three markers used most frequently in the clinical practice are basal FSH, antral follicle count (AFC), and anti-Müllerian hormone (AMH) levels.

1.2.1.1 Early Follicular Follicle-Stimulating Hormone Levels (Basal FSH)

Early follicular phase serum FSH levels are inversely correlated with the number of follicles in the ovary as determined histologically. It is important to mention that it should always be measured with basal estradiol levels. Higher day 3 FSH positively correlates with the age of patients and negatively with the estradiol (E_2) response to stimulation and the number of oocytes retrieved, though it was found that basal FSH testing is limited by wide intercycle variability, which weakens its reliability (5–7). Basal FSH may serve as a predictor of decreased ovarian response, and an abnormally high basal FSH value has a high predictive value for decreased ovarian response. However, a normal value has a low negative predictive value for poor response. In addition, basal FSH has no value in predicting OHSS.

Although basal FSH level as a predictive marker has marked shortcomings, it is clear that the pregnancy and live birth rates declined with increasing FSH and advancing age, confirming the importance of utilization of age-specific FSH levels in assessing infertile women (8). For patients with FSH receptor defect, the basal FSH levels are elevated, but other ovarian reserve markers (AFC and AMH) are normal or even high.

1.2.1.2 Antral Follicle Count (AFC)

The ovary contains three distinct populations of developing follicles: primordial follicles, early-growing follicles, and antral follicles. A small proportion of early-growing follicles develop into antral follicles larger than 2 mm. These are highly responsive to FSH and can be readily visualized using transvaginal ultrasound. AFC is typically carried out at the beginning of a cycle, counting those small antral follicles between 2 and 8 mm. However, recent evidence suggests that AFC can be obtained at any point in the cycle without compromising accuracy, and with the recent development of three-dimensional ultrasound and other improvements in ultrasound resolution, antral follicles as small as 2 mm in diameter can now be reliably counted.

For several important IVF outcomes, AFC has been associated with good predictive value, showing a linear relationship with the number of retrieved oocytes and correlation with measures of ovarian response to gonadotrophins, including cycle cancellations as a result of poor response. However, it did not predict implantation rate, pregnancy rate, or live birth rate. Presently, AFC is an easy-to-perform, noninvasive approach that immediately provides essential predictive information on ovarian responsiveness, both low and hyperresponse, with acceptable interoperator reliability (9) (Table 1.1).

1.2.1.3 Anti-Müllerian Hormone (AMH)

AMH is a transforming growth factor-b superfamily member, secreted exclusively from ovarian granulosa cells by primary and secondary preantral (but not primordial) and small antral follicles (up to 5–6 mm). Through paracrine mediation, AMH contributes to control follicle development from the reserve of primordial follicles constituted early in life, and its production seems to be independent of FSH. Its serum levels positively correlate with histologically determined primordial follicle number and negatively correlate with chronologic age.

During the last few years, AMH has emerged as one of the most important clinical markers for ovarian reserve in assisted reproductive techniques (ART). It has a strong correlation with the number of follicles, it is operator independent, it can predict reproductive life-span, and it is useful as a baseline assessment preceding ovarian stimulation for individualizing the therapeutic strategy. AMH levels are associated with ovarian response, becoming an excellent predictor of poor ovarian response, excessive response, and pregnancy outcomes in IVF (10).

The main limitation of AMH is the presence of significant biological intra- and intercycle variation, as we will discuss below, and the assay methods. Due to dissimilarity in the antibodies and assay sensitivities, in addition to interlaboratory variations, a considerable difference has been found between different assays, particularly for low AMH values, making their interpretation complicated. Furthermore, the presence of different AMH isoforms not detectable with most of the assays reduces the accuracy of the results. The highly sensitive, fully automated AMH assays that have been available since 2014 have replaced the older ELISA assays, thereby both providing faster results and improving interobserver reliability. However, no reliable converting factor has been identified; therefore, the cut points developed and reported for one commercial AMH assay are not generalizable to others (6, 10) (Table 1.1).

1.2.2   Variability of the Ovarian Reserve Test

Ovarian reserve tests have three main goals (Summary 1.1): [1] counseling IVF patients based on ovarian response prediction and the probability of live birth; [2] employing predicted ovarian response to optimize ovarian stimulation and minimize safety risks; and [3] assessing current and future fertility potential to allow women to decide when and how to proceed with family planning, fertility treatment, or fertility preservation. The ideal ovarian reserve test should be convenient; be reproducible; display little, if any, intracycle and intercycle variability; demonstrate high specificity to minimize the risk of wrongly diagnosing women as having diminished ovarian reserve; and accurately identify those at greatest risk of developing ovarian hyperstimulation prior to fertility treatment. An ovarian reserve measure without limitations has not yet been discovered, although both AFC and AMH have good predictive value and clearly have an added value together with female age and basal FSH for predicting ovarian response in IVF (6). Unfortunately, still today (anno 2019), there is a lack of studies combining the BMI to the aforementioned ovarian reserve markers, in order to have a more objective assessment of the patient's response.

AMH has been considered an ovarian reserve marker that can be measured independently of the cycle phase with minimal fluctuations in the menstrual cycle. Initially, those fluctuations were associated with the analysis, as analytical variability. It is true that different platforms will deliver different results depending on which molecular form of AMH is being measured, sample storage, freezing of samples, the assay protocols, and manual or automated methods used. However, recent studies have revealed inter- and intracycle variations that cannot be explained only by analytical variability, underlying the presence of a biologic AMH dynamic that is not yet fully understood. During the natural cycle, serum AMH levels

---

Summary 1.1 Evaluation of Ovarian Reserve

Ovarian Reserve Marker Goals

1. To counsel patients based on ovarian response prediction and live birth rate
2. To optimize ovarian stimulation and minimize safety risks
3. To assess current and future fertility potential for family planning

The Ideal Ovarian Reserve Test

- Convenient for the patient
- Reproducible
- Little intracycle and intercycle variability
- Accurate to identify patients who will have poor response or hyperresponse

Table 1.1 AFC versus AMH: Pros and cons

AFC	AMH
• Easy to perform • Noninvasive • Provides immediate results • To be carried out at the beginning of a cycle because of intracycle variation • Interoperator variation observed	• Well characterized across adolescent and reproductive ages • Analytical variability depending on the assays and sample storage • No standardization across assays • Faster results available with the fully automated assays
• Both markers have good predictive value for the number of oocytes retrieved and stimulation response. • Both are helpful to guide protocol and other treatment decisions. • Physicians need to be aware of intracycle and intercycle variability.	

seem to be higher during the follicular phase than the luteal phase, and recently, our group described a 20 percent intraindividual AMH variability during the ovarian cycle, using a fully automated AMH assay. As well, we observed 28 percent of short-term intercycle variations, probably caused by a biological variation in the number of AMH-producing antral follicles, since those follicles, due to their size, produce a significant amount of AMH. Similarly, when the intercycle variation of AFC was examined, cycle-to-cycle measurements revealed only moderate agreement in any range of counts due to the variable size of the growing follicle cohort among separate cycles. These observations may explain the intercycle variations of the ovarian response for the same patient when the same stimulation protocol is used. Hence, fluctuations in the same woman, intercycle and intracycle during natural cycles, question whether a single AMH or AFC measurement is enough for decision-making in our daily practice (10, 11).

1.2.3 The Best Moment to Measure AMH

Nowadays, it seems clear that AMH can fluctuate during the menstrual cycle with not only intracycle but also short-term intercycle variations that cannot be explained by the AMH assaying. As well, this happens with AFC. This variability should be considered carefully before making any decision in assisted reproductive technologies.

Hence, when should AMH and AFC be used?

Based on their variations shown during the whole cycle, it would be useful during our daily work to standardize the moment for the evaluation, as the results for our patients will be more homogeneous. As a routine, we perform the AFC during the first days of the cycle before starting the ovarian stimulation, so we visualize by ultrasound the follicles that would be expected to respond to the medication. This information is combined with the basal AMH levels on days 1–3 of the cycle, measured with automated assay (Elecsys, Roche). With both ovarian reserve markers and AMH and AFC during the early follicular phase, combined with the patient's age and basal FSH, more accurate information is obtained for the ovarian stimulation prognosis, and the dosage of medication for each patient is adjusted based on the results.

1.3 Ovarian Response Classification: The Cutoff Values

An important factor when using ovarian reserve markers as predictors of ovarian response is to establish acceptable cutoff levels, values that can distinguish with sufficient accuracy women who are likely to have normal responses from those likely to have abnormal responses to ovarian stimulation. AMH and AFC values reported in literature are very variable (cutoff levels of AMH values for poor ovarian response have been reported between 0.1 and 2.97 ng/mL, which is within the range of normal values for AMH in healthy women), thus creating difficulties for clinicians in selecting the best cutoff values based on evidence (12).

The lack of a uniform definition of a poor response makes it difficult to compare studies and challenging to develop or assess any protocol to improve the outcome. In 2011, a consensus was reached to standardize the definition of poor ovarian response (POR) in a reproducible manner: the Bologna Criteria. These include at least two of the following three features: (1) advanced maternal age or any other risk factor for poor ovarian response (POR); (2) a previous POR; and (3) an abnormal ovarian reserve test (ORT). Two episodes of POR after maximal stimulation are sufficient to define a patient as a poor responder in the absence of advanced maternal age or abnormal ORT. A low or poor ovarian response was considered to be the retrieval of three or fewer oocytes (Summary 1.2) (13).

Conversely, a hyperresponse (or high response) is often defined as the retrieval of 15–20 or more oocytes and is associated with an exponential increase in the risk of ovarian hyperstimulation syndrome (OHSS). Henceforth, a normal response would be in between both.

In a recent publication in the Cochrane Database, Lensen et al. (14) used the following cutoffs to guide the categorization of women using markers of ovarian reserve:

- AMH < 7 pmol/L, AFC < 7, bFSH > 10 IU/L categorized as predicted low responders
- AMH 7 pmol/L to 21 pmol/L, AFC 7 to 15 categorized as predicted normal responders (bFSH is not considered to be a reliable predictor for normal response)
- AMH > 21 pmol/L, AFC > 15 categorized as predicted high responders (bFSH is not considered to be a reliable predictor for hyperresponse)

However, the limits between low and normal response, and between normal and high response, are difficult to define accurately. We prefer to consider that there is a gray area of transition between one category to the other. For these patients with ovarian reserve markers in between categories, the individualization of doses will make the difference: adequate dosage would maximize the success rate, minimizing the treatment burden or the OHSS risk (Figure 1.1) (12).

1.4 Individualization: Initial Doses and Dose Adaptation

Although personalization of IVF treatment may lead to an improvement in patient compliance and better clinical practice, it is far from easy. The difficulty derives not only from the vast number of drugs and choices available for controlled ovarian stimulation (COS) but, as well, from the best cycle to start the treatment for a given patient, when and how to trigger for final oocyte maturation, and the best approach to plan embryo transfer.

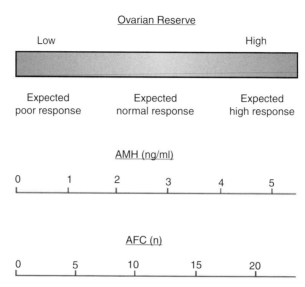

Figure 1.1 Ovarian reserve testing before the first IVF cycle would permit to categorize patients as expected poor, normal, or hyperresponders. The limits between low and normal response, and between normal and high response, are difficult to define accurately. Adequate dosage would maximize the success rate, minimizing the treatment burden or the OHSS risk. From La Marca et al. (12), with permission. A black and white version of this figure will appear in some formats. For the colour version, please refer to the plate section.

Summary 1.2 Poor Ovarian Response as per Bologna Criteria

At least two of the following three features must be present:

- Advanced maternal age (≥40 years) or any other risk factor for POR
- A previous POR (≤ three oocytes with a conventional stimulation protocol)
- An abnormal ovarian reserve test (i.e., AFC: five to seven follicles or AMH: 0.5–1.1 ng/mL)

Two episodes of POR after maximal stimulation are sufficient to define a patient as a poor responder in the absence of advanced maternal age or abnormal ORT.

1.4.1 Gonadotropin Dosage: What Is the Optimal Number of Oocytes to Obtain?

A major challenge in IVF treatment represents the selection of the most adequate dosage of medication for a sufficient ovarian response. However, the first step should be to reach an agreement regarding the optimal outcome of ovarian stimulation in terms of the number of oocytes being retrieved.

Taking into account the increasing use of embryo freezing and the significant progress in cryopreservation techniques, including vitrification, cumulative live birth rate (LBR) appears to be considered a more complete measure of success of an IVF treatment; in this context, the optimal number of oocytes retrieved needs to be

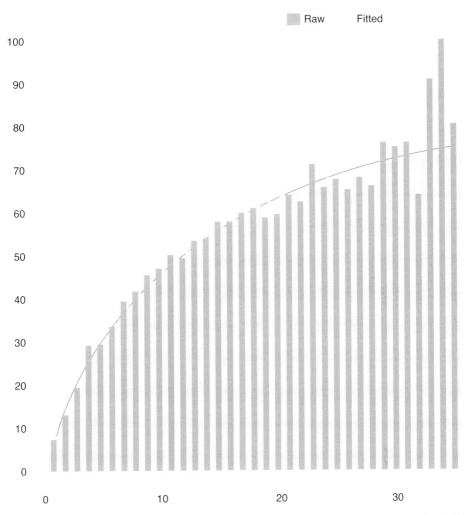

Figure 1.2 Cumulative LBRs according to the number of oocytes: observed (raw) versus predicted (fitted) probability. LBRs continuously increase with the number of oocytes retrieved. From Polyzos et al. (15), with permission.

determined in terms of cumulative LBR. Recently, a retrospective multicenter cohort study conducted in 15 hospitals in Europe (15) correlated the cumulative LBR and the number of oocytes retrieved for more than 14,000 patients who performed IVF/ICSI with GnRH antagonist protocol. Based on its results, cumulative LBRs do not reach a plateau and continuously increase with the number of oocytes retrieved, with a moderate increment beyond 27 oocytes (Figure 1.2). This steady increase is evident in all age categories, with lower cumulative LBRs with increasing age for a given number of eggs. However, OHSS rates are considerably higher in women with >25 oocytes in the case of fresh ET, as expected. Furthermore, accumulating evidence involving genetic analysis for aneuploidy screening has clearly demonstrated an increase in the number of euploid embryos with the number of oocytes retrieved (16–18). The final total number of euploid embryos is the most meaningful outcome, explaining the increased cumulative LBR in the higher oocyte categories.

Therefore, in the era of vitrification, cumulative LBRs continuously increase with the number of oocytes retrieved (19). Nevertheless, although very high ovarian response may further increase cumulative LBRs, ovarian stimulation should be rational and avoid extreme response in terms of oocytes retrieved to preserve patients' convenience and safety and avoid OHSS or other iatrogenic complications. Moreover, the response is directly linked with the change of steroids, which may also have a negative impact on the endometrium and oocyte quality, if the gonadotropin dose is not adjusted toward the end of the follicular phase, according to patient response (3).

1.4.2 High Responders

In predicted high responders, as described above, we should balance between optimal ovarian stimulation with successful treatment outcomes and minimal rates of moderate/severe OHSS. We should combine different strategies for this purpose, and reducing the doses of FSH for ovarian stimulation is only one of them. Individualization of treatments, elective single embryo transfer, and the option of freezing all embryos replacing hCG with GnRH agonist (GnRHa) triggers may further reduce the incidence of OHSS. As well, the use of different medications after the egg retrieval, such as cabergoline, letrozole, or GnRH antagonist, will reduce further the incidence of early OHSS (13).

1.4.3 To Program the Cycle: To Pill or Not to Pill

Worldwide, gonadotrophin-releasing hormone (GnRH) antagonists are gaining ground, and the number of patients being treated for IVF with a GnRH antagonist is increasing. For these protocols, synchronization of follicular cohort is an important factor for the success of the stimulation. Moreover, cycle planning has also been a challenge in GnRH antagonist cycles. During the past few years, debates have been ongoing about the possible disadvantages of oral contraceptive pill (OCP) pretreatment in GnRH antagonist IVF cycles, and some publications describe that OCP pretreatment might have a negative effect on outcome in GnRH antagonist IVF cycles. However, when patients received the pill for only 12–16 days and had a wash-out period of at least 5 days, no differences could be found in live birth rates. Moreover, when cycles planned with OCP were compared with cycles pretreated with estrogens only, again, no differences could be found in live birth rates.

The benefits of cycle scheduling with the pill, such as synchronization of follicular cohort, must be weighed against the drawbacks (i.e., higher FSH consumption and longer duration of the stimulation). If given for a minimum number of days and initiation ovarian stimulation after a wash-out period that resembles the natural cycle, OCP pretreatment might not have a negative effect on endometrial receptivity, and IVF outcome might be comparable to that in women undergoing a classical long protocol or who were pretreated only with estrogens (20).

1.4.4 Dose Adaptation during Stimulation

A receptive endometrium depends on the interaction of the hormones estrogen and progesterone and is crucial to allow embryo implantation. Endometrial receptivity is driven by progesterone exposure after sufficient estrogen exposure and is obviously at stake when progesterone elevation occurs during the late follicular phase of ovarian stimulation for IVF. Progesterone level increases with the size of follicular diameter, and in ovarian stimulation for IVF with a large number of growing follicles, each follicle will contribute to the progesterone in the systemic circulation. Under the influence of progesterone, the histological appearance of the endometrium changes. Compared with natural cycles, a more advanced secretory endometrial maturation is found in stimulated cycles, and additionally, using a cutoff level of 1.5 ng/mL for elevated progesterone levels on the day of HCG administration, there is an alteration of the endometrial gene expression patterns. This situation leads to reduced pregnancy rates when the embryo transfer is carried out in the same cycle. Furthermore, several recent studies also suggest an impairment of oocyte and embryo quality. The causes of premature progesterone elevation during ovarian stimulation are still unclear; however, recently published data point toward the fact that enhanced FSH stimulation toward the end of the follicular phase might be the primary cause for progesterone elevation (21).

To avoid the negative effect of elevated progesterone levels on the implantation rate and subsequently on the pregnancy rate, different strategies could be considered: first, individualization of stimulation dosage according to the patient's ovarian reserve. Second, the incidence of progesterone elevation can be lowered by reducing the gonadotropin dose toward the late follicular phase of ovarian stimulation according to the patient's response (21, 22) (Figure 1.3). Third, in the event of progesterone elevation on the day of trigger, fresh embryo transfer should not be carried out and cycle segmentation should be applied. The "freeze-all" approach with a subsequent transfer of the embryos in a natural or hormonal replacement cycle eliminates the detrimental effect of elevated progesterone levels on the endometrial receptivity (23) (Summary 1.3).

1.4.5 The Trigger for the Final Oocyte Maturation

Once the correct gonadotropin dose, based on patients ovarian reserve parameters has been calculated and administered, and the gonadotropin dose has been adapted toward the end of the follicular phase, based on the individual patients response, also the final oocyte maturation can be and should be individualized, according to the patients' requirements. The type and dosage of medication, and how many hours prior the oocyte retrieval, will make the difference in the final number of mature eggs retrieved. This decision should be based in different factors: the ovarian reserve markers, patient BMI, the use of OCP during the previous cycle, the hormonal levels at the beginning and at the end of the stimulation, and the number of follicles seen by US before the trigger.

Following GnRH antagonist co-treatment during ovarian stimulation, final oocyte maturation at the end of the follicular phase can also be induced by a bolus dose of a GnRH agonist generating a relative short endogenous LH (and FSH) surge, partially mimicking a natural ovulation. For high responders, this approach will reduce drastically the risk of OHSS. However, the levels of endogenous FSH and

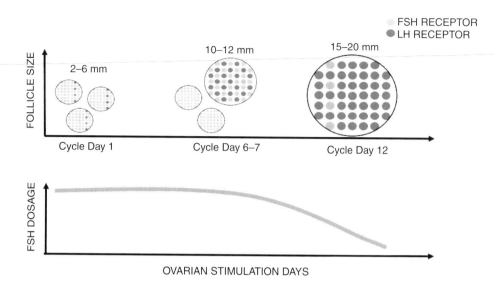

Figure 1.3 Follicle development and FSH/LH receptor expression during the ovarian stimulation. FSH receptors are predominant during the early follicular phase and have a steady reduction as the follicle increases in size and maturity (25). LH receptors are predominant at the late follicular phase. To reduce the incidence of progesterone elevation, the gonadotropin dose should be slowly reduced toward the late follicular phase, according to the patient's response, with no detrimental effect on follicle growth (21, 22). A black and white version of this figure will appear in some formats. For the colour version, please refer to the plate section.

Summary 1.3 Rescue Strategies to Prevent Premature Rise of Progesterone and Actions to Take If Progesterone Elevation Cannot Be Avoided

- Avoidance of enhanced ovarian stimulation toward the end of the follicular phase by performing a step-down approach reduces the incidence of P elevation on the day of final oocyte maturation.
- Prolonging ovarian stimulation should be avoided, as it will increase the risk of P elevation.
- A freeze-all approach with performance of the embryo transfer in a subsequent cycle. The impact of P elevation on the endometrium will be eliminated completely.

Today, the prevention of premature P elevation is essential as elevated P levels on the day of final oocyte maturation are associated with reduced pregnancy rates. Individualization of ovarian stimulation treatment includes choosing the correct stimulation dosage according to the patient's ovarian reserve parameters and to adapt the stimulation dosage according to the hormonal levels during ovarian stimulation.

LH rise will be associated with the rate of mature oocytes retrieved and may result in an inadequate oocyte yield in a small subset of patients. This failure can range from empty follicle syndrome to the retrieval of much fewer oocytes than expected. It has been shown that patients with immeasurable LH levels on trigger day have an up to

25 percent risk of suboptimal response. Patients with immeasurable LH levels at the start of stimulation (<0.1 IU/l) had a 45.2 percent risk of suboptimal response, while the risk decreased with increasing basal LH levels. LH values should be measured prior to start of ovarian stimulation. In cases where suboptimal response to GnRH agonist trigger can be anticipated, an individualized approach is warranted (24).

Another reason for suboptimal response after the trigger for final maturation is obesity. For patients with high body mass index (BMI), subcutaneous administration may end with suboptimal absorption and, therefore, suboptimal results. In such cases, intramuscular administration of hCG or intranasal administration of GnRH agonist will improve the rate of mature oocytes retrieved.

When GnRH agonist triggering for final oocyte maturation is performed, and the decision is taken for a fresh embryo transfer, luteal phase supplementation with low-dose hCG, based on luteal coasting (see Chapter 4) should be considered.

1.5 Conclusions

The way to approach any patients for an ART treatment should be fully personalized. Individualization of treatment is not new to the field of medicine, although this concept is relatively fresh in reproductive medicine, and still is generating controversies. The availability of new markers of ovarian reserve, the improvement in methodology for their measurement and the huge amount of clinical data have supported the view that individualization in IVF is the way forward. Age, FSH, AFC, and AMH have an important role in the prediction of the ovarian response and for enabling the subsequent individualization of a therapeutic strategy. This is the basis for the correct selection of the different GnRH analogs and, for the fine-tuning of the gonadotrophin dose. Subsequently, the adjustment of the stimulation dosage during late follicular phase according to the patient's response and the final triggering for oocyte maturation will further increase the chances to obtain mature oocytes.

References

1. Doody K, Griesinger G, Witjes H, et al. High ovarian response does not jeopardize ongoing pregnancy rates and increases cumulative pregnancy rates in a GnRH-antagonist protocol. Hum Reprod 2013;28(2):442–452. doi:10.1093/humrep/des389.

2. Sunkara SK, Rittenberg V, Raine-Fenning N, et al. Association between the number of eggs and live birth in IVF treatment: an analysis of 400 135 treatment cycles. Hum Reprod 2011;26:1768–1774.

3. Lawrenz B, Labarta E, Fatemi H, et al. Premature progesterone elevation: targets and rescue strategies. Fertil Steril 2018;109 (4):577–582. doi:10.1016/j.fertnstert.2018.02.128.

4. Mourad S, Brown J, Farquhar C. Interventions for the prevention of OHSS in ART cycles: an overview of Cochrane reviews. Cochrane Database Syst Rev 2017;1: CD012103.

5. Muasher SJ, Oehninger S, Simonetti S, et al. The value of basal and/or stimulated serum gonadotropin levels in prediction of stimulation response and in vitro fertilization outcome. Fertil Steril 1988;50:298–307.

6. Niederberger C, Pellicer A, Cohen J, et al. Forty years of IVF. Fertil Steril 2018;15 (2):185–324e5. doi:10.1016/j.fertnstert.2018.06.005.

7. Broekmans FJ, Kwee J, Hendriks DJ, et al. A systematic review of tests predicting ovarian reserve and IVF outcome. Hum Reprod Update 2006;12:685–718.

8. Gleicher N, Kushnir VA, Sen A, et al. Definition by FSH, AMH and embryo numbers of good-, intermediate- and poor-prognosis patients suggests previously unknown IVF outcome-determining factor associated with AMH. J Transl Med 2016;14:172. doi:10.1186/s12967-016-0924-7.

9. Fleming R, Seifer D, Frattarelli J, et al. Assessing ovarian response: antral follicle count versus anti-Müllerian hormone. Reprod BioMed Online 2015;31:486–496. doi:10.1016/j.rbmo.2015.06.015.

10. Melado L, Lawrenz B, Bungum L, et al. Anti-Müllerian hormone variability during ovarian stimulation for IVF: a novel approach to predict fertility treatment outcomes. J Reprod Biol Endocrinol 2018;2(1):33–34.

11. Melado L, Lawrenz B, Sibal J, et al. Anti-Müllerian hormone during natural cycle presents significant intra and intercycle variations when measured with fully automated assay. Front Endocrinol 2018;9:686. doi:10.3389/fendo.2018.00686.

12. La Marca A, Sunkara SK. Individualization of controlled ovarian stimulation in IVF using ovarian reserve markers: from theory to practice. Hum Reprod Update 2014;1:124–140. doi:10.1093/humupd/dmt037.

13. Ferraretti A, La Marca A, Fauser BCJM, et al. ESHRE consensus on the definition of "poor response" to ovarian stimulation for in vitro fertilization: the Bologna criteria. Hum Reprod 2011;26(7):1616–1624.

14. Lensen SF, Wilkinson J, Leijdekkers JA, et al. Individualised gonadotropin dose selection using markers of ovarian reserve for women undergoing in vitro fertilisation plus intracytoplasmic sperm injection (IVF/ICSI). Cochrane Database Syst Rev 2018;2:CD012693. doi:10.1002/14651858.CD012693.pub2.

15. Polyzos NP, Drakopoulos P, Parra J, et al. Cumulative live birth rates according to the number of oocytes retrieved after the first ovarian stimulation for in vitro fertilization/intracytoplasmic sperm injection: a multicenter multinational analysis including ~15,000 women. Fertil Steril 2018;110(4):661–670. doi:10.1016/j.fertnstert.2018.04.039.

16. Orvieto R, Vanni VS, Gleicher N. The myths surrounding mild stimulation in vitro fertilization (IVF). Reprod Biol Endocrinol 2017;15(1):48. doi:10.1186/s12958-017-0266-1.

17. Labarta E, Bosch E, Alama P, et al. Moderate ovarian stimulation does not increase the incidence of human embryo chromosomal abnormalities in in vitro fertilization cycles. J Clin Endocrinol Metab 2012;97:1987–1994.

18. Gleicher N, Kim A, Weghofer A, et al. Lessons from elective in vitro fertilization (IVF) in, principally, non-infertile women. Reprod Biol Endocrinol 2012;10:48.

19. Fatemi HM, Doody K, Griesinger G, et al. High ovarian response does not jeopardize ongoing pregnancy rates and increases cumulative pregnancy rates in a GnRH-antagonist protocol. Hum Reprod 2013;28:442–452. doi:10.1093/humrep/des389.

20. García-Velasco JA, Fatemi HM. To pill or not to pill in GnRH antagonist cycles: that is the question! Reprod Biomed Online 2015;30(1):39–42. doi:10.1016/j.rbmo.2014.09.010.

21. Lawrenz B, Beligotti F, Engelmann N, et al. Impact of gonadotropin type on progesterone elevation during ovarian stimulation in GnRH antagonist cycles. Hum Reprod 2016;31:2554–2560.

22. Lawrenz B, Fatemi H. Effect of progesterone elevation in follicular phase of IVF-cycles on the endometrial receptivity. Reprod Biomed Online 2017;34:422–428.

23. Fatemi HM, García-Velasco JA. Avoiding ovarian hyperstimulation syndrome with the use of gonadotropin-releasing hormone agonist trigger. Fertil Steril 2015;103:870–873.

24. Popovic-Todorovic B, Santos-Ribeiro S, Drakopoulos P, et al. Predicting suboptimal oocyte yield following GnRH agonist trigger by measuring serum LH at the start of ovarian stimulation. Hum Reprod 2019;27. doi:10.1093/humrep/dez132.

25. Jeppesen JV, Kristensen SG, Nielsen ME, et al. LH-receptor gene expression in human granulosa and cumulus cells from antral and preovulatory follicles. J Clin Endocrinol Metab 2012;97(8):E1524–1531. doi:10.1210/jc.2012-1427.

Individualized Ovarian Stimulation in Patients with Advanced Maternal Age and Premature Ovarian Aging

Norbert Gleicher and David H. Barad

2.1 Introduction

Because studies of older and, otherwise, unfavorable patients going through in vitro fertilization (IVF) treatments with their own (autologous) oocytes are sparse, we here present to a large degree the subjective experience of only one fertility center in New York City, which as of this point contributed a majority of published studies on this subject. As US national IVF data registries by the Center for Disease Control and Prevention (CDC) and the Society for Assisted Reproductive Technologies (SART) demonstrate, *this center* serves the by-far oldest patient population among over 500 reporting US IVF centers and, therefore, likely the oldest patient population of any IVF center in the world. While the median age of all US centers reporting to the *CDC* in 2016 was 36 years, this center's median age was 42 years in 2016 and 43 years in 2017 and 2018. Over 90 percent of the center's new patients in recent years reported prior failed IVF cycles, often at multiple centers. Over half of the center's patients are so-called long-distance patients from outside the larger New York City Tri-State area, many from Canada and overseas. Finally, in excess of 95 percent of the center's patients suffer from LFOR, which means that even younger patients usually demonstrate abnormally high age-specific follicle-stimulating hormone (FSH) and abnormally low anti-Müllerian hormone (AMH). This center, thus, overall, likely, serves the poorest-prognosis patient population of any IVF center in the world.

This chapter describes in detail the treatment of such poor-prognosis patients. Poor response to ovarian stimulation is a very subjective diagnosis: It can be caused by many treatment-independent factors, like wrong medication dosing, poor quality medications, poor absorption of medications, or patient errors. The definition of poor response also changes with advancing age. We, therefore, do not favor the diagnostic terminology of "poor response," as expressed by the Bologna Criteria (1) and, instead, prefer to define patients objectively by their functional ovarian reserve (FOR), also called the growing follicle pool (Box 2.1). Objectively poor responders, will usually, of course, demonstrate LFOR. These two patient definitions, therefore, to a degree overlap. Utilizing the idiom

NG and DHB are listed as co-owners of a number of already awarded and still pending US patents, some claiming benefits from androgen supplementation in women with low ovarian reserve, a topic peripherally addressed in this manuscript. NG is a shareholder in Fertility Nutraceuticals LLC, which produces a DHEA product, and is owner of The CHR. NG and DHB receive patent royalties from Fertility Nutraceuticals LLC. NG and DHB also received research support, travel funding, and lecture fees from various pharma and medical device companies, none, in any way, related to this manuscript.

Box 2.1 Definition of Ovarian Reserve (OR) Components

OR is the sum of all follicles/oocytes a woman has left over at any given age. OR, therefore, declines with advancing age. OR is made up of two distinct components:

The larger part is represented by the so-called resting pool of primordial follicles, which cannot be directly assessed, and the so-called growing follicle pool, represented by all follicles after recruitment between primary follicle stage and small preantral stages. The size of the growing pool can be assessed with FSH, AMH, and antral follicle counts (AFCs), though correlations are not perfect. Size of the growing pool, indirectly, also defines the resting pool because both pools are proportional in size. Because the growing follicle pool defines ovarian function, we also call it the FOR. Abnormally high age-specific FSH and/or low AMH denote LFOR, while abnormally high age-specific AMH in many cases denotes a diagnosis of polycystic ovary syndrome (PCOS), even though international PCOS criteria, still, do not include AMH in the definition of PCOS.

LFOR, rather than poor response as diagnostic term, also offers the opportunity of a prospective diagnosis, while poor response always represents a postfactum diagnosis after a usually unsatisfactory IVF cycle.

All over the world, but especially in the more developed countries, infertility patients are aging. As a consequence, donor egg cycles have been surging. Despite significantly lower pregnancy chances, most women, however, still prefer their own eggs over donor eggs. Demand for autologous cycles is, therefore, increasing. Considering the very substantial changes with advancing female age in ovarian physiology, one would assume appropriate adjustments in IVF treatments of older women. Likely because the literature on the subject has remained so sparse, such adjustments are, however, only rarely made.

The same argument also applies to women with premature ovarian aging (POA), also called occult primary ovarian insufficiency (oPOI), which in many features mimics ovarian aging. Younger women with POA/oPOI, therefore, often require similar treatments as older women (2). Both of these patient groups in the medical literature frequently are combined under acronyms, like poor/low responders, LFOR, or poor-prognosis patients. They share a need for individualized treatments, which this chapter will attempt to describe.

2.1.1 Background

As women are, likely, born with all of their eggs. OR represents all remaining follicles/eggs a woman still maintains in her ovaries. OR, thus, declines with advancing age. It is made up of resting follicles, also called primordial follicles, and the so-called growing follicles after recruitment from the resting pool. We here describe the growing follicle pool as a patient's FOR because the resting pool is not available to clinical interventions (Box 2.1).

For the longest time, the growing follicle pool was also considered outside of therapeutic reach. Infertility practice, indeed, over the last 60 years concentrated practically exclusively only on the last two weeks of follicle maturation, the so-called gonadotropin-dependent stage of follicle maturation, when follicles become sensitive to gonadotropin stimulation. Only during those two weeks, do follicles respond to traditional fertility medications, including exogenously administered gonadotropins. By the time follicles reach this developmental stage, it, however, appears reasonable to assume that most of a follicle's fate has already been determined. That during those two weeks effects on egg and, therefore, embryo quality at most will only be marginal, has in recent years been increasingly recognized and, likely, represents a main contributing factor why over 40 years the concept of "embryo selection" has only been marginally successful at best.

An underreported conceptual breakthrough, however, occurred over 10 years ago, when the importance of appropriate androgen levels for follicle maturation became apparent in animal models at small-growing follicle stages (3) and in concomitant clinical androgen supplementation studies (4). Though by some still considered a controversial issue (5), what has been widely overlooked is the fact that androgen supplementation of selected infertile women represented in 60 years of modern infertility treatment the first extension of fertility treatments from the last two weeks of follicle maturation in the gonadotropin-dependent stage into earlier stages of folliculogenesis.

With the oocyte believed to contribute ca. 95 percent of embryo quality, the importance of this revolutionary step for modern infertility care cannot be overemphasized because, the more upstream interventions occur, the more will they beneficially impact oocyte quality and, ultimately, embryo quality. An important goal of modern infertility research, therefore, must be to switch from 40 years of, understandably, not very successful attempts at embryo selection, toward attempting to improve embryo quality through interventions into earlier stages of recruitment and oocyte maturation.

Observations surrounding androgen supplementation of selected infertile women also significantly contributed to a better understanding of what, likely, represents ovarian aging. There is consensus that ovarian aging concomitantly means a number of different things: With advancing age, women, for example, persistently lose follicles/oocytes. How many follicles/oocytes a woman's ovaries still contain, therefore, defines her "ovarian age." In ca. 90 percent of women, chronological and ovarian ages are the same; in the remaining 10 percent, however, remaining follicles/oocytes numbers are below normal. So-affected women are generally described to suffer from POA/oPOI and, as will be further discussed in more detail below, clinically and physiologically, they often behave like much older women.

Ovarian aging is, however, not only a quantitative but also a qualitative problem. Remarkably, even if age, AMH and FSH are controlled for, and if identical numbers of embryos are transferred, infertile women with progressively more embryos available for transfer will demonstrate progressively better and better pregnancy and live birth chances in IVF until a peak in AMH levels is reached, implantation rates start to reverse and miscarriage rates progressively increase (6). Until this AMH peak is reached (at usually very high levels), quantity and quality of oocytes and embryos, therefore, usually coincide, except in one only recently described condition, the so-called hypoandrogenic PCOS-like phenotype (H-PCOS) (7, 8), further discussed below.

Traditionally, with advancing female age, declining egg quality has been linked to the natural aging process of primordial follicles in ovaries. Though aging of primordial follicles, not only quantitatively but, likely, also qualitatively, plays an important part in ovarian aging, the center's experience with androgen supplementation led to a revised hypothesis. It proposes that, due to the almost complete isolation of primitive primordial follicles from their surrounding stroma, aging-induced environmental damage on primordial follicles over time is only limited. Good evidence in support can be found in the observation that some even highly toxic chemotherapeutic agents do not damage primordial follicles (9), while others, of course, do (10). Once recruited into small-growing follicle stages, follicles, however, almost uniformly are severely damaged by chemo- as well as radiation therapy and undergo apoptosis.

This new ovarian aging hypothesis builds on these observations by making the argument that primordial follicles cannot be too badly damaged by advanced female age if, postrecruitment, androgen supplementation can still significantly improve IVF cycle outcomes (4). Like chemotherapy damage, at least some age-dependent damage to follicles, therefore, must happen postrecruitment. Assuming this, indeed, to be the case, this damage to follicles/oocytes must happen postrecruitment, at early stages of follicle maturation, and not prerecruitment at primordial stages, as current dogma holds. Granulosa cells of small-growing follicle stages are characterized by greatest density of androgen receptors (Figure 2.1) (3, 4). The culprit, therefore, must be the ovarian microenvironment in which these maturation stages take place: a hypoandrogenic ovarian microenvironment.

This new hypothesis of ovarian aging, therefore, not only explains how androgen supplementation can beneficially affect female infertility but opens the field to much wider potential treatment horizons in establishing that oocyte quality can be beneficially affected through early intervention into folliculogenesis (in itself, a major innovation in the treatment of female infertility) and, second, by concentrating research efforts on the ovarian microenvironment of older ovaries.

If treatment of androgen deficiencies can lead to better egg quality, there must be innumerable, yet to be discovered, additional deficiencies in the ovarian microenvironment that occur with advancing female age. Further improvements in the ovarian microenvironment can, therefore, be expected to yield similar incremental improvements, witnessed with androgen supplementation (4). Within this context, it is also of interest

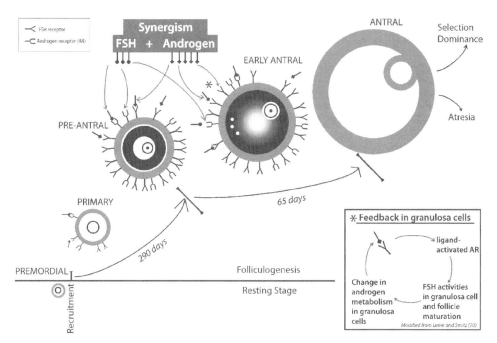

Figure 2.1 FSH and androgen receptors during small-growing follicle stages. Modified from Gleicher et al. (13), with permission. A black and white version of this figure will appear in some formats. For the colour version, please refer to the plate section.

that worldwide popularity of human growth hormone (HGH) supplementation in IVF cycles has recently significantly increased, even though HGH may only increase oocyte yields, without improving pregnancy and live birth chances (11). Achieving its effectiveness via IGF-1, HGH, like androgens, primarily improves FSH activity on granulosa cells at small-growing follicle stages.

Follicles enter the growing follicle pool after recruitment and require at least additional 6–8 weeks to reach the gonadotropin-dependent stage, where they become available to exogenous gonadotropin stimulation in IVF cycles. Appropriate timing of supplementation of the ovarian microenvironment is, therefore, crucial: Exerting effects primarily at small-growing follicle stages (Figure 2.1), supplementation of androgens and HGH must, therefore, be started at least 6–8 weeks prior to IVF cycle start (12, 13). If supplementation is offered only during IVF cycles (as, unfortunately, is practice at many IVF centers), follicles stimulated in that cycle will get hardly any benefits, though recent reports raised the possibility of positive androgen and HGH supplementation effects also on the implantation process (14, 15).

2.1.2 How to Select Patients for Individualized Fertility Treatments

For decades, most IVF centers have been following specific treatment protocols, which only rarely diverge from established baselines. To maintain consistency of results, such an approach made sense, as long as patient populations were relatively cohesive. With IVF outcomes till ca. 2010 steadily improving (16), initially uniform patient populations started, however, increasingly to diverge into better- and poorer-prognosis patients. Better-prognosis patients conceived quicker, thus rapidly exiting fertility treatments. Poorer-prognosis patients, however, lingered and, over time, increased in absolute numbers as well as in proportions of total patients in treatment.

Poorer-prognosis patients were mostly older women, desirous of conceptions at ever-increasing ages, but also younger women with POA/oPOI and, therefore, almost equally poor pregnancy and live birth chances. Both of these patient populations were in obvious need of distinctively different treatment algorithms and more individualized infertility treatments. In many treatment aspects both groups also overlapped and, therefore, shared the fate of, often, being given no choice but third-party egg donation cycles rather than individualized cycles with autologous oocytes. The IVF field, therefore, largely missed out on the rapidly evolving concept of "personalized medicine" that swept medical practice in most specialty areas over the last decade. This kind of individualized personalized medicine is, however, exactly what is required if the dramatic declines in live birth rates observed all over the world since 2010 (16, 17) are to be reversed.

Though these developments seemed too obvious to be overlooked, they did not lead to reassessments of mostly uniform and universal protocols in favor of more individualized approaches, but to rapidly growing utilization of third-party egg donation cycles, which, indeed, in 2010 in parallel with live birth rates peaked (16, 17). As a consequence, the IVF field really never learned to treat poor-prognosis patients with individualized treatment protocols because most, instead, ended up in third-party donor egg cycles.

Returning to our preferred patient classification of good, average, and poor prognoses based on age-specific FOR, female patients can at all ages be classified into these categories quite easily. The reason is in IVF's above noted almost universal interdependence of quantity and quality of oocyte yields. Embryo numbers available for transfer, therefore, ultimately determines prognosis (6). But FOR is, of course, age-dependent and declines as women age. What represents a favorable FOR, associated with good prognosis, therefore, also changes, as do determinations of average and poor prognoses.

FOR is clinically traditionally determined through FSH, AMH and in some centers via antral follicle counts (AFCs). Theoretically, they should correlate, but some distinct differences exist. Many centers, for example, consider AFCs a more subjective FOR parameter than FSH and AMH levels and, therefore, do not use them as objective parameters in daily patient assessments. Others, on the other hand, use AFCs as primary assessment tools in order to avoid blood draws. Also, at extremely low levels, AMH loses its clinical predictability, while evaluations of FSH are, of course, cycle-day-dependent (should be drawn on days 2/3 of cycle) and easily influenced by estradiol levels (FSH, therefore, must be drawn in association with estradiol).

A study performed a number of years ago investigated various FSH/AMH combinations and their respective outcomes in clinical IVF practice (18). Surprisingly, best pregnancies were achieved in women with high-FSH/high-AMH patterns. When originally reported, the authors had no good explanation for these findings. They, however, since, were able to explain them after discovering a new diagnostic entity in infertile women (named H-PCOS; see below for further detail) (7, 8). Though FSH and AMH in general correlate in the inverse, there are exceptions with potentially significant diagnostic relevance.

Since FOR changes with age, FSH, AMH, and AFC must be evaluated in age-specific ways. Remarkably, this, however, happens only in a small minority of IVF centers. IVF practitioners who do not consider FSH, AMH, and/or AFCs in age-specific ways will fail to diagnose in timely fashion those with abnormally LFOR in POA/oPOI and older patients or those with excessively high FOR – mostly cases of PCOS.

Since many laboratories consider FSH levels up to 10.0 or even 12.0 mIU/mL as "normal range," many women with POA/oPOI do not necessarily present with "abnormal" FSH. For example, an FSH of 9.9 mIU/mL in a 25-year-old cannot be considered normal, even if still in "normal" laboratory range. The same level in a 46-year-old, on the other hand, may actually denote unusually good FOR considering her age. In reverse, an AMH of 1.0 ng/mL at age 25 is strongly suggestive of POA/oPOI but at age 45 would actually denote exceptionally good FOR.

Table 2.1 summarizes diagnoses mandating special attention and, therefore, individualized IVF protocols. As already noted, one population that automatically qualifies are women of advanced age. Because in early IVF days, age 38 represented the upper age limit for IVF treatments, advanced female age has in association with IVF historically been defined as age above 38 years. With improved abilities to achieve pregnancies in older women, the definition of advanced female age moved to age 40. Based on contemporary IVF practice, in which women above age 42 are mostly referred into third-party egg donations (16, 17), it can now be considered to start at roughly age 42.

Though in the US IVF with autologous oocytes is rare above age 42–43, we have been advocating treatments of older women with autologous oocytes with the argument that outcomes can be better than has been widely perceived (19). Outcomes, of course, cannot approach treatment successes achieved with young third-party donor eggs. Genetic maternity does, however, represent a principal desire and goal of most female infertility patients, and must be respected under a patient's right to self-determination.

Young women with POA/oPOI, as previously noted, mimic older women in many physiologic as well as clinical observations. Consequently, treatments often are quite

Table 2.1 Infertility diagnoses, warranting individualized IVF care

Diagnoses	Main features
Advancedage	•Age above 38, but especially above 42, even with normal age-specific FOR
POA/oPOI	•Low age-specific FOR
	•Hypoandrogenic
	•Often associated with autoimmunity
POF/POI (age <40) or early menopause (40–50)	•Menopausal FOR
	•Hypoandrogenic
	•Often associated with autoimmunity
PCOS	•Often associated with immune system hyperactivity (inflammation, autoimmunity)
	•FOR is age-dependent but generally excessive
Classical phenotype	•Abnormally high age-specific FOR at all ages
	•Hyperandrogenic at all ages with peripheral manifestations (hirsutism, acne, etc.)
	•Truncal obesity
	•Frequent anovulation
Lean phenotype (here also called H-PCOS) (7, 8)	•FOR variable depending on androgen levels but AMH often high in relation to FSH
	•Hyperandrogenic in teens and early 20s, followed by drop to hypoandrogenism
	•Rare peripheral manifestations
	•Lean
	•Rare anovulation in teens and early 20s only

Note. FOR, functional ovarian reserve, also called the growing follicle pool; hypoandrogenism reflects low testosterone levels [lower third of normal range in association with elevated sex hormone binding globulin (SHBG)]; POA/oPOI, premature ovarian aging/occult primary ovarian insufficiency; POF/POI, premature ovarian failure/primary ovarian insufficiency; PCOS, polycystic ovary syndrome.

similar. Because diagnostic terminologies can at times be confusing, a clear understanding of which patient populations should be given specific treatments is of utmost importance. So, for example, a recent systematic review in a reputable medical journal claimed to address pregnancy following premature ovarian insufficiency (20). It further defined this condition by criteria of the European Society of Human Reproduction and Embryology (ESHRE) as primary or secondary amenorrhea for more than 4 months, onset before age 40 and FSH over 25 mIU/mL (21). One of the two references the authors cited, however, referred to a diagnosis of *primary* rather than *premature* ovarian insufficiency (22), a more commonly used terminology. Though both terminologies can be abbreviated as POI and are defined by similar criteria, they are substantially different because primary ovarian insufficiency is defined by FSH levels above 40.0 mIU/mL, rather than 25 mIU/mL (23).

This is a crucially important differentiation because POA/oPOI, the precursor condition to POI, is often defined by abnormally elevated FSH between 10.0 and 12.0 mIU/ml up to 40.0 mIU (though, as noted before, should really be determined in age-specific ways). Premature ovarian insufficiency, as defined in the above-referenced review and by ESHRE criteria, is, therefore, a very different condition from POI, a distinction, unfortunately, lost in the above-cited review and in much of the infertility literature. Box 2.2 defines terminologies, and with it, patient populations, as they are described in this chapter.

Individualization of treatments is obviously dependent on accurate and consistent differential diagnoses between precursor and full ovarian insufficiency. A clear understanding of here used terminology is, therefore, of importance. Women with POF/POI (menopausal FOR before age 40), or with simply early physiologic menopause between ages 40 and 51–52 years, are obviously distinct in their respective therapeutic interventions from POA/oPOI patients, even though they may share underlying etiologies (24).

LFOR usually produces abnormally low oocyte yields in IVF (i.e., so-affected women exhibit ovarian resistance to stimulation with gonadotropins). Conditions with abnormally high FOR, in contrast, result in unusually large egg numbers for age and, therefore, often create risks of ovarian hyperstimulation. In an overwhelming number of cases, they represent PCOS patients, with classical and lean phenotypes, combined, representing somewhere between 80 and 90 percent of cases. In contrast to the classical phenotype, the lean phenotype often goes undiagnosed, a subject this chapter will return to later.

Extremes of ovarian response and ovarian function are, therefore, defined by POA/oPOI and POF/POI at the low and PCOS at the high end. Neither extreme represents, however, homogenous patient populations. Both, therefore, require highly individualized care, even though reasons, of course, differ. Especially at younger ages, large egg numbers, for example, automatically denote increased risk for ovarian hyperstimulation and ovarian hyperstimulation syndrome (OHSS), a potentially life-threatening complication of IVF.

PCOS has remained controversial since it does not represent one distinct diagnosis but, likely, a basket of conditions. A detailed review of PCOS would exceed the framework of this

---

Box 2.2 Terminology of Ovarian Failure Diagnoses Used in This Chapter

Terminologies used in the medical literature in describing ovarian insufficiency are very confusing and at times contradictory. To be precinct in presentation of materials in this chapter, we, therefore, want to be very clear in describing patient populations to which reference is made: Premature ovarian aging (POA), also called occult primary ovarian insufficiency (oPOI) (23), involves women below age 40 with abnormally LFOR, as demonstrated by elevated age-specific FSH up to a maximum level of 40.0 mIU/mL and/or abnormally low age-specific AMH. Once FSH levels are persistently above 40.0 mIU, the patient is still under age 40 and is amenorrheic, her diagnosis is primary ovarian insufficiency (POI), also called premature ovarian failure (POF). Once patients exhibit the POI/POF phenotype but at time of diagnosis are older than age 40, their diagnosis is early menopause. Physiologic menopause occurs at median age of 51–52 years. Secondary ovarian insufficiency (SOI) or failure (SOF) occurs when ovaries become insufficient due to inadequate adrenal androgen levels, which inhibits follicle maturation at small-growing follicle stages immediately after recruitment (3, 4).

chapter; therefore, only so much: Different clinical presentations of PCOS, based on international consensus, have been described as "phenotypes," with the "classical" and the "lean" phenotypes representing over 80 percent of all cases, each reflecting ca. 40 percent of the PCOS population.

When contemplating PCOS, because of the very typical appearance of this phenotype, even most physicians, however, only imagine the classical PCOS phenotype, characterized by hyperandrogenism, truncal obesity, short stature, anovulation and oligo-amenorrhea, hirsutism, acne, and development of the metabolic syndrome later in life. The lean pheno-type, in contrast, are women who look entirely normal and have none of above noted stigmata of the "classical" phenotype, are usually ovulatory and have regular menstrual patterns (Table 2.2). Like classical phenotypes, they, however, in their teens, are hyperan-drogenic and may encounter rare short-term menstrual irregularities. Investigating the ontogeny of this phenotype (7, 8), the possibility was raised that this phenotype represents the continuum of the nodular adrenal hyperplasia described by the Stratakis laboratory at the National institutes of Health (NIH) (25). Because the lean PCOS phenotype is rather unremarkable in its clinical presentation, it is frequently overlooked, and patients are often classified as "unexplained" in their infertility.

The only characteristics classical and lean phenotypes share are high androgen levels at younger years (teens to mid-20s) and, persistently into advanced ages, abnormally high

Table 2.2 Characteristics of the hypoandrogenic PCOS-like phenotype

- Diagnosis can be reached at all ages
- AMH high for age
    - disproportionate to FSH (high FSH/high AMH) (18)
- Large age-disproportionate egg numbers in prior IVF cycles
- Poor egg/embryo quality (i.e., quantity/quality discrepancy)
- High androgens in teens to mid-20s
- Rapid decline in androgens between mid-20s and mid-30s
- Low androgens   for age after ~35
    - low free and total testosterone
    - DHEA/DHEAS > 2/1[a]

- Relatively high SHBG
- Cortisol   mildly high in teens to mid-20s[a]
    - mildly low after age 35

- Evidence of autoimmunity in ca. 85% of cases
    - Thyroid autoimmunity in ca. 45% of cases

Note. AMH, anti-Müllerian hormone; FSH, follicle-stimulating hormone; DHEA, dehydroepian-drosterone; SHBG, sex hormone binding globulin.

[a] Since low testosterone levels are usually associated with low DHEAS, the observed hypoandrogenism is likely of adrenal rather than ovarian origin. Because insufficiencies of the other two zonae of the adrenals are autoimmune in nature and because H-PCOS is so highly associated with autoimmune findings in general, investigators assumed that H-PCOS was an autoimmune condition of the adrenals which, because of the resulting hypoandrogenism, adversely affects ovarian function, leading to a form of secondary OI (SOI). Possibly representing the nodular adrenal hyperplasia reported by Gougari et al. (25) in teenagers.

AMH levels for age. Since classical and lean PCOS patients quite often present with mildly elevated FSH levels, they often present with the previously noted high FSH/high AMH pattern. In contrast to classical PCOS, the lean PCOS phenotype, however, loses its hyperandrogenism in the age range of 25–35 years, starting in the mid-30s a typical endocrine pattern of persistently high AMH but, in contrast to classical PCOS, low androgen levels (and, therefore, often high SHBG). Because international bodies do not yet recognize elevated AMH in the diagnosis of PCOS, women with this presentation have been given the diagnosis of the hypoandrogenic PCOS-like phenotype (H-PCOS) (7, 8).

Professional consensus for the longest time has been that, clinically, the classical PCOS was the more "unfavorable" phenotype to have. To a degree, this argument still holds, but this is the case only because patients are phenotypically so severely affected and later in life suffer from metabolic syndrome. Regarding infertility, lean PCOS has, however, surprisingly been found to be the more difficult one to succeed with. This was discovered as investigators attempted to research the ontogeny of PCOS with advancing female age. To everybody's surprise, in extracting PCOS patients from the center's anonymized electronic patient database, the researchers discovered that the center basically exclusively served "lean" PCOS patients (26). As a center of last resort for most patients who previously underwent IVF treatments elsewhere, the only explanation for this discovery was that classical PCOS patients conceived before reaching this center, while lean PCOS patients apparently did not.

Investigating the "lean" PCOS phenotype further, investigators then were able to define its characteristics, its above briefly described ontogeny and even hypothesize about its etiology (7, 8). It, indeed, in principle encompasses what under Rotterdam Criteria has been described as the lean PCOS phenotype. Table 2.2 summarizes its characteristics. Once well defined, its prevalence among patients was found to be surprisingly high.

As H-PCOS patients became better understood, it became apparent that older H-PCOS patients who already developed hypoandrogenism, in analogy to POA/oPOI patients, required androgen supplementation before IVF cycle start if their egg and embryo quality was to be improved and, with it, their pregnancy chances. Patient diagnosed with H-PCOS are, therefore, routinely supplemented with DHEA.

These observations also, finally, offered an explanation for previously noted study of FSH/AMH pairings that discovered high FSH/high AMH to produce best pregnancy chances in association with IVF, an unexplained finding at that time (18). The center then already routinely supplemented fertility patients with low androgens with DHEA. Unknowingly, that had included women with at that point still unknown H-PCOS, which fairly typically presented with discrepant FSH and AMH, level, the unusual combination of high FSH and high AMH, low androgens, and elevated SHBG (Table 2.2). Up to that point treatment-resistant at other IVF centers, supplemented with DHEA, these patients experience the center's highest IVF pregnancy rates, explaining previously unexplained findings in the original publication (18).

2.2 Individualized Treatments

After describing in the preceding section which patients represent the most important potential subjects for individualized fertility treatments, we in this section describe what those individualized treatments entail. In recognition of almost all fertility patients preferring to conceive with autologous oocytes, the context remains a treatment philosophy that considers third-party egg donations, strictly, only last resort treatments, though fully recognizing and communicating to patients that, in practically all cases, pregnancy and live birth chances with autologous oocytes will be significantly inferior to donor eggs. Ultimate treatment choices are, however, always the patients', with clear understanding that physicians have the absolute obligation of presenting all available treatment options to patients with unvarnished outcome prospects but are not qualified to tell patients how to live their lives.

In practical terms this philosophy means that treatment choices are always left to patients, even if their choices contradict recommendations made by physicians. In recognition that the decision to turn toward third-party egg donation represents a highly complex and very personal decision and that patients, therefore, should not be pushed, or even forced into such a decision, a patient's treatment choice should never be refused, unless it carries with it significant risks to the patient's health. This philosophy is also based on the recognition how important certainty is for many women (and often also their partners) that they, indeed, are unable to conceive with use of their own eggs before choosing third-party egg donation.

2.2.1 Preparation of Ovaries

Not *yet* being able to produce "new" oocytes for women with either LFOR and/or with poor quality oocytes, the concept of pretreating ovaries prior to IVF cycle start has been gaining. Though many colleagues still believe that oocyte quality is fixed and unassailable, as previously explained, evidence suggests otherwise: With the microenvironment of ovaries aging, crucially important components for follicle maturation within this microenvironment are becoming deficient. Androgens and IGF-1/HGH are the only such components so far identified. It seems logical that essential components of the ovarian microenvironment, now lacking in appropriate concentrations, be replenished. Such replenishments, moreover, must occur in timely fashion.

When it comes to supplementation of androgens and IGF-1/HGH, that time point is the small-growing follicle stage immediately after recruitment, which means that supplementation must be initiated at least 6–8 weeks before IVF cycle start. Such presupplementation of IVF cycles appears essential because of the time it takes for the so-treated follicles to reach gonadotropin-dependency and become sensitive to the effects of exogenous gonadotropin stimulation. Older women above age 40, POA/oPOI, POF/POI (27), and more recently as reported above, H-PCOS patients (7, 8), have all been identified as women in need of androgen presupplementation.

Since the human body produces testosterone from DHEA, such supplementation via DHEA (25 mg TID, p.o. Fertility Nutraceuticals LLC). Every organ in the body capable of producing testosterone will in this way take up only as much DHEA as it needs to achieve desired testosterone levels (and testosterone levels vary between human organs). Though testosterone can also be administered directly, its administration via patch or transdermal gel floods the whole body, with every organ getting equal amounts. Side effects of direct testosterone administration are, therefore, somewhat more pronounced. Moreover, risk of reaching toxic testosterone levels for reproductive success, with DHEA supplementation minimal, are significantly higher with testosterone.

Because of a large number of animal models that not only demonstrated the importance of androgens for normal follicle maturation but also demonstrated beneficial effects from supplementation of low androgen levels (3, 4), even in absence of adequately powered prospectively randomized studies, androgen supplementation can be considered an adequately established treatment modality. The same, however, cannot be said about HGH presupplementation, which we still consider experimental and, currently, investigate in a prospectively randomized study in which patients receive 3–6 IU of HGH (various manufacturers) daily for 8 weeks prior to IVF cycle start.

In addition to prenatal vitamins, poor-prognosis patients also receive supplementation with CoQ10, depending on absorption characteristics at 600–1000 mg daily. In mice, this antioxidant has been found effective in improving egg quality and quality of cumulus cells (28, 29). Though human data for such effectiveness are lacking, considering its relative low cost and lack of side effects, we consider supplementation with CoQ10 in poor-prognosis patients advisable. From research in other medical specialty areas, this antioxidant is known to improve mitochondrial function in human cells (30). With the mature egg being the largest cell in the female body, also carrying the largest mitochondrial load, supplementation prior to IVF cycle start appears to make sense.

2.2.2 Ovarian Stimulation

How to stimulate poor-prognosis patients with LFOR is more an issue of what *not* to do in ovarian stimulation, rather than how to stimulate correctly. So, for example, since after age, the number of good-quality embryos available for embryo transfer is the second-most important predictor of pregnancy and live birth chances (6), we do not understand the arguments made in the literature for mild stimulation cycles or even natural cycles. We, therefore, stimulate such patients aggressively, which uniformly means stimulation with a mixture of FSH (350–450 I.U.) and hMG (150 I.U.) per day.

Another stimulation feature that must be avoided is ovarian suppression. In women of advanced age and in other poor-prognosis patients with LFOR, we avoid hormonal contraceptives and full-dose agonists and antagonists, and, if prevention of premature spontaneous ovulation is required, that is achieved with the microdose agonist protocol initially reported by Surrey et al. (31).

Recognizing that premature luteinization of the follicular microenvironment accelerates with advancing female age as well as in women with POA/oPOI (32, 33), the need for such microdose agonist protocols has, however, at our center in the last five years greatly diminished due to increasing utilization of highly individualized egg retrieval (HIER), described in the next paragraph.

2.2.3 Highly Individualized Egg Retrieval (HIER)

Luteinization of mature follicles is a normal occurrence. Relatively recently acquired knowledge, however, suggests that, as women age, onset of premature luteinization in follicles occurs earlier and earlier (32, 33). Consequently, retrievals of oocytes at all (ovarian) ages at the same leading follicle sizes will in older women and some younger patients with POA/oPOI lead to premature follicle luteinization, representing a toxic environment for mature oocytes (at *CHR* jokingly called "hard-boiled" in place of "soft-boiled" eggs). With follicles and oocyte undergoing speeded up maturation, retrieval timing must be adjusted. Table 2.3 summarizes ranges of lead follicle sizes based on female age. Here listed lead follicle sizes, at recommended hCG trigger of 10,000 IU, are only age-dependent ranges. Other factors within each age group must also be considered when determining lead follicle size for hCG trigger at cycle start. For example, a 45-year-old woman with undetectable AMH and only 1–2 follicles on ultrasound, will have to be approached differently from a 45-year-old patient with 15 follicles and an AMH of 3.9 ng/mL. Individualization of timing of hCG administration is, therefore, of crucial importance. This is where the term HIER comes from, indicating the importance of highly individualized timing of the hCG trigger that establishes oocyte retrieval timing.

Table 2.3 Lead follicle ranges with HIER at different female ages

Lead follicle size at hCG administration (10,000 IU)	
Standard retrieval	19–22 mm
POA/oPOI mild	16–18 mm
Severe	14–16 mm
Above age 40 years	
40–42 years	16–18 mm
43–45 years	14–16 mm
>45 years	12–14 mm
>48 years	<12 mm

When HIER was first introduced into clinical practice, all cycles were triggered at 16 mm lead follicle size, and we were surprised how low the rate of immature MI and especially GV oocytes was. At the same time, we, however, noticed that a considerable number of oocytes were still atretic and that this number increased with advancing age. This observation led to the conclusion that 16 mm lead follicle size could not remain the lower limit. The oldest reported patient to conceive and deliver a child with use of autologous oocytes at our center and in the world was, indeed, triggered at 12 mm, ca. two weeks short of her forty-eighth birthday (19).

2.2.4 Treatments of Associated Conditions

Older infertility patients and younger women with LFOR often suffer from associated medical conditions. As women are getting older, all medical conditions, indeed, increase in prevalence. For that reason, once they conceive, poor-prognosis patients in fertility clinics usually are also defined as high-risk obstetric patients.

A few conditions, however, are deserving of special considerations and, among those, the likely most important one, yet frequently still overlooked, is what in most general terms can be described as *elevated miscarriage risk*. Older women are, of course, at increased miscarriage risk, simply because of their increased aneuploidy rates at advanced ages. That, however, does not mean that every miscarriage in an older woman must, automatically, be viewed as age-related and, therefore, as chromosomal. Autoimmunity also increases with age, as do uterine abnormalities, especially myomas.

Younger women with POA/oPOI represent the highest risk for miscarriages (34) and also demonstrate a high degree of autoimmune abnormalities (24). When treating poor-prognosis patients, it, therefore, is not only enough to help them conceive; one must also keep in mind that many of those same patients also need help staying pregnant.

Because of limited remaining time for conception, pregnancy losses are much more devastating for older than younger women. Especially if pregnancy losses occur relatively late in pregnancy (as is the case with autoimmunity, while chromosomal losses usually occur relatively early), older patients not only mourn loss of pregnancy but also wasted time in, often last-ditch efforts, to conceive with autologous oocytes. In attempts to maximize prevention, treatments of poor-prognosis patients, therefore, must prophylactically attempt to discover increased miscarriage risks to avoid potentially preventable pregnancy losses.

2.3 Conclusions and the Future

We hope here to demonstrate that, based on their right to self-determination, older women and other poorer-prognosis patients have the absolute right to choose utilization of their own eggs over donor eggs, even though young donor eggs usually offer much better pregnancy and live birth chances. We also hope to have demonstrated here why, and how certain, new stimulation-related treatments are beneficial to poorer-prognosis patients, while the withholding of other treatments, especially treatments with suppressive effects on ovaries, is recommended. We also strongly believe that extended culture-to-blastocyst stage is generally contraindicated in poorer-prognosis patients and transfers at cleavage stage are preferable. Similarly, we oppose mild stimulation and natural cycle IVF, since egg and embryo numbers are highly predictive of IVF outcomes at all ages. The more transferrable embryos a cycle yields, not only are cumulative pregnancy rates higher but implantation rates for embryos are also higher at all ages (6).

We also oppose other "fashions of the moment," add-ons to IVF, made mostly since ca. 2010 (16, 17), when IVF live birth rates peaked around the world. Largely manufactured for revenue rather than clinical purposes, they in timing have been highly associated with dramatic declines in pregnancy and live birth rates since 2010 and usually have been brought to market without prior validation studies. As preimplantation genetic testing for aneuploidy (PGD-A) well demonstrates, poor-prognosis patients are usually the most vulnerable to adverse outcome effects in association with IVF (35, 36) since they can least afford inadvertent losses of eggs, embryos, or anything else that potentially translates into additional pregnancy chances (35).

Not all is bad in the field, however, because we live in an era of extraordinary discovery in basic embryology with not only enormous potential implications for reproductive medicine but for medicine in many other specialty areas as well. For what appears on the horizon, the reader is referred to a recent article (36). Expected changes to fertility treatments can be expected to be revolutionary rather than evolutionary, and will radically affect what is currently considered standard practice.

References

1. Ferraretti AP, La Marca A, Fauser BC, et al. ESHRE working group on Poor Ovarian Response Definition. ESHRE consensus on the definition of "poor response" to ovarian stimulation for in vitro fertilization: the Bologna criteria. Hum Reprod 2011;26 (7):1616–1624.

2. Gleicher N, Weghofer A, Barad DH. Defining ovarian reserve to better understand ovarian aging. Reprod Biol Endocrinol 2011;7(9):23.

3. Sen A, Hammes SR. Granulosa cell-specific androgen receptors are critical regulators of ovarian development and function. Mol Endocrinol 2010;24(7):1393–1403.

4. Prizant H, Gleicher N, Sen A. Androgen actions in the ovary: balance is key. J Endocrinol 2014;222(3):R141–151.

5. Montoya-Botero P, Rodriguez-Purata J, Polyzos NP. Androgen supplementation in assisted reproduction: where are we in 2019? Curr Opin Obstet Gynecol 2019;31 (3):188–119.

6. Gleicher N, Kushnir VA, Sen A, et al. Definition by FSH, AMH and embryo numbers of good-, intermediate- and poor-prognosis patients suggests previously unknown IVF outcome-determining factor associated with AMH. J Transl Med 2016;14 (1):172.

7. Gleicher N, Kushnir VA, Darmon SK, et al. New PCOS-like phenotype in older infertile

women of likely autoimmune adrenal etiology with high AMH but low androgens. J Steroid Biochem Mol Biol 2017;167:144–152.

8. Gleicher N, Kushnir VA, Darmon SK, et al. Suspected ontogeny of a recently described hypo-androgenic PCOS-like phenotype with advancing age. Endocrine 2018;59 (3):661–676.

9. Stringer JM, Swindells EOK, Zerafa N, et al. Multidose 5-fluorouracil is highly toxic to growing ovarian follicles in mice. Toxicol Sci 2018;166(1):97–107.

10. Nguyen QN, Zerafa N, Liew SH, et al. Cisplatin- and cyclophosphamide-induced primordial follicle depletion is caused by direct damage to oocytes. Mol Hum Reprod 2019. doi:10.1093/molehr/gaz020. [Epub ahead of print]

11. Norman RJ, Alvino H, Hull LM, et al. Human growth hormone for poor responders: a randomized placebo-controlled trial provides no evidence for improved live birth rate. Reprod Biomed Online 2019;38 (6):908–915.

12. Gleicher N, Barad DH. Dehydroepiandrosterone (DHEA) supplementation in diminished ovarian reserve (DOR). Reprod Biol Endocrinol 2011;9:67.

13. Gleicher N, Weghofer A, Barad DH. The role of androgens in follicle maturation and ovulation induction: friend or foe of infertility treatment? Reprod Biol Endocrinol 2011;17(9):116.

14. Gibson DA, Simitsidellis I, Kelepouri O, et al. Dehydroepiandrosterone enhances decidualization in women of advanced reproductive age. Fertil Steril 2018;109 (4):728–734.

15. Cui N, Li AM, Luo ZY, et al. Effects of growth hormone on pregnancy rates of patients with thin endometrium. J Endocrinol Invest 2019;42(1):27–35.

16. Gleicher N, Kushnir VA, Barad DH. Worldwide decline of IVF birth rates and its probable causes. Hum Reprod Open 2019;2019(3):hoz017.

17. Gleicher N, Barad DH. IVF practice changes after 2010 are associated with lowest IVF live birth rates since 1990. [In review]

18. Gleicher N, Kim A, Kushnir V, et al. Clinical relevance of combined FSH and AMH observations in infertile women. J Clin Endocrinol Metab 2013;98 (5):2136–2145.

19. Gleicher N, Kushnir VA, Darmon S, et al. Older women using their own eggs? Issue framed the issue with two oldest reported IVF pregnancies and a live birth. Reprod Biomed Online 2018;37(2):172–177.

20. Fraison E, Crawford G, Casper G, et al. Pregnancy following diagnosis of premature ovarian insufficiency: a systematic review. Reprod Biomed Online 2019. doi:10.1016/ jrbmo.2019.04.019.

21. Webber L, Davies M, Anderson R, et al. ESHRE Giodeline: management of women with premature ovarian insufficiency. Hum Reprod 2016;31:926–937.

22. Baber R. Primary ovarian insufficiency. Med Today 2014;15:73–75.

23. Nelson LM. Clinical practice: primary ovarian insufficiency. N Engl J Med 2009;360(6):606–614.

24. Gleicher N, Weghofer A, Oktay K, et al. Do etiologies of premature ovarian aging (POA) mimic those of premature ovarian failure (POF)? Hum Reprod 2009;24 (10):2395–2400.

25. Gougari E, Lodish M, Keil M, et al. Bilateral adrenal hyperplasia as a possible mechanism for hyperandrogenism in women with polycystic ovary syndrome. J Clin Endocrinol Metab 2016;101 (9):3353–3360.

26. Kushnir VA, Halevy N, Barad DH, et al. Relative importance of AMH and androgens changes with aging among non-obese women with polycystic ovary syndrome. J Ovarian Res 2015;9(8):45.

27. Gleicher N, Kim A, Weghofer A, et al. Hypoandrogenism in association with diminished functional ovarian reserve. Hum Reprod 2013;28(4):1084–1091.

28. Ben-Meir A, Burstein E, Borrego-Alvarez A, et al. Coenzyme Q10 restores oocyte mitochondrial function and fertility during reproductive age. Aging Cell 2015;14 (5):887–895.

29. Ben-Meir A, Kim K, McQuaid R, et al. Co-enzyme Q10 supplementation rescues cumulus cells dysfunction in a maternal aging model. Antioxidants (Basel) 2019;8(3):58.

30. Luo K, Yu JH, Quan Y, et al. Therapeutic potential of coenzyme Q_{10} in mitochondrial dysfunction during tacrolimus-induced beta cell injury. Sci Rep 2019;29(91):7995.

31. Surrey ES, Bower J, Hill DM, et al. Clinical and endocrine effects of a microdose GnRH agonist flare regimen administered to poor responders who are undergoing in vitro fertilization. Fertil Steril 1998;69(3):419–424.

32. Wu YG, Barad DH, Kushnir VA, et al. Aging-related premature luteinization of granulosa cells is avoided by early oocyte retrieval. J Endocrinol 2015;226 (3):167–180.

33. Wu YG, Barad DH, Kushnir VA, et al. With low ovarian reserve, highly individualized egg retrieval (HIER) improves IVF results by avoiding premature luteinization. J Ovarian Res 2018;11(1):23.

34. Levi AJ, Raynault MF, Bergh PA, et al. Reproductive outcome in patients with diminished ovarian reserve. Fertil Steril 2001;76(4):666–669.

35. Mastenbroek S, Twisk M, van Echten-Arends J, et al. In vitro fertilization with preimplantation genetic screening. N Engl J Med 2007;357 (1):9–17.

36. Gleicher N. Expected advances in human fertility treatments and their likely translational consequences. J Transl Med 2018;16(1):149.

Individualized Oocyte Maturation

Gustavo Nardini Cecchino, Diego Ventura Tarasconi, and
Juan Antonio García Velasco

3.1 Introduction

In vitro fertilization (IVF) outcomes are strongly correlated with the number of mature oocytes retrieved following controlled ovarian stimulation (COS) (1). Cumulative live birth rates continuously increase with the number of oocytes available, irrespective of the patient's age (2). Multiple factors may influence the number of oocytes to be fertilized, such as the use of individualized stimulation protocols, patient compliance, and the ovulation trigger (OT) strategy.

In natural cycles, the processes of follicle dominance and oocyte maturation rely on the shift of follicular FSH-dependency to LH-dependency, as the FSH levels fall along the end of the follicular phase leading to atresia of nondominant follicles (3). The FSH activity is responsible for nuclear maturation, induction of LH receptors in granulosa cells and maintenance of cumulus cell-to-cell communication. It also stimulates the conversion of plasminogen into plasmin protease that will provoke the rupture of the follicular wall before ovulation (4, 5). Conversely, the LH peak will initiate the ovulatory cascade by promoting the resumption of the meiosis in oocytes and luteinization of the granulosa cells, which will result in reduced estrogen levels and increased progesterone and prostaglandins secretion, essential for follicle rupture (6).

In stimulated cycles with exogenous gonadotropins, final oocyte maturation can only be achieved after artificial induction of a LH surge with GnRH agonist (GnRHa) or through the administration of human chorionic gonadotropin (hCG), which will act directly on LH receptors. In IVF cycles, ovulation is usually triggered when at least two follicles reach 17–18 mm in mean diameter, or the serum estradiol levels are compatible with 200–300 pg/mL per follicle in the final stage of development. Finally, oocyte retrieval is performed 34–36 h after OT.

A synchronous maturation of both the nucleus and the cytoplasm of the oocyte is crucial to yield top-quality embryos. Oocyte maturity is determined by the expansion of the cumulus mass, radiance of corona cells, the size and cohesiveness of granulosa cells as well as the shape and color of the oocyte (7). Nuclear maturation involves germinal vesicle breakdown, normally induced by the LH surge, followed by resumption of meiosis and, ultimately, extrusion of the first polar body (7).

A mature oocyte must be in the metaphase II stage (MII) of the second meiotic division. The final oocyte maturation is achieved after the resumption of the meiosis promoted by the hormonal surge of gonadotropins, either in natural or stimulated cycles (7). Furthermore, the ability of an oocyte to resume and complete meiosis is also related to the mean follicular diameter (8). Up to 30–40 percent of the oocytes are usually immature at the time of retrieval following COS, which reflects the varying size of the follicles at the time of the ovulation trigger (8). An oocyte retrieval can be considered optimal when more than 75 percent of the oocytes obtained are in the MII stage (9).

3.2 Triggering Ovulation in IVF Cycles

There are different OT strategies that may be used in IVF cycles. In order to reach the best maturity rate, an optimized OT strategy must be applied taking into account the type of ovarian stimulation protocol, the type of OT agent, and the timing of the oocyte pick-up after the trigger. Different scenarios deserve a personalized OT approach and clinical decision-making will vary according to the baseline characteristics of patients, response to COS, and embryo transfer schedule.

Theoretically, ovulation may be triggered with distinct agents, such as recombinant LH, kisspeptin, hCG, and GnRHa (10). However, in daily clinical practice only hCG and GnRHa are used. The current formulation of the recombinant LH (75 IU/vial) makes it unpractical to reach the 30,000 IU needed to induce ovulation (11). Regarding the kisspeptin, there is lack of consistent evidence (9, 10).

3.2.1 hCG Trigger

There is no specific receptor for hCG, but its pharmacological structure and biological similarity to LH, allow it to bind to the LH receptors (LHCG-R) and induce ovulation in gonadotropin-stimulated cycles (12). The first evidence on the existence of a LH/hCG receptor was demonstrated several decades ago, by *in vitro* studies using rat Leydig cells (13). These experiments found similar sets of binding sites and binding capacity for both hormones. Due to the additional 30 amino acids at its unique beta subunit, hCG binding has longer half-life, during approximately 7 days (14). Such a sustained luteotropic activity could lead to severe side effects through the release of vasoactive substances (e.g., vascular EGF) and prostaglandins (Figure 3.1) (10).

There are two forms of hCG available: a) hCG extracted from the urine of pregnant woman or placental tissue, which is less pure; b) recombinant hCG produced with biomolecular technologies offering high purity and consistency. There are issues regarding the potency and dose equivalency of recombinant versus urinary hCG, but most studies indicate that 250 ug of the recombinant product is comparable with 5,000 to 10,000 UI of the urinary one (15). The most recent Cochrane review and meta-analysis failed to demonstrate any

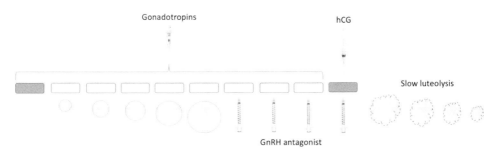

Figure 3.1 hCG trigger. Slow luteolysis offers an adequate luteal phase support. A black and white version of this figure will appear in some formats. For the colour version, please refer to the plate section.

difference in reproductive outcomes and ovarian hyperstimulation syndrome (OHSS) incidence between the use of urinary and recombinant hCG for OT (15).

3.2.2 GnRHa Trigger

The use of GnRH agonist to induce an endogenous LH surge sufficient to trigger ovulation in IVF cycles was first described in 1990 (16). This strategy can only be applied in IVF cycles using a GnRH antagonist-induced downregulation or progestin priming, because of the competitiveness for the same receptor. Due to its greater affinity for the GnRH receptor than the endogenous GnRH, a bolus of agonist will promote a "flare-up" of gonadotropins, enough to induce final oocyte maturation with a much shorter duration than hCG (Figure 3.2) (17).

Despite the lower LH serum levels following the use of GnRHa, the concomitant release of FSH may add further physiological benefits and reduce adverse events such as OHSS (18). First reports using GnRHa revealed worst reproductive results most likely due to an insufficient luteal phase support after the "flare-up" period (19, 20). Adequate luteal phase support proved to improve outcomes (21). To date, neither large retrospective studies nor randomized clinical trials found significant differences between GnRH agonist trigger and hCG in terms of reproductive outcomes. Considering the faster drop in gonadotropins concentration along with desensitization and blockage of the receptor, appropriate luteal phase support must be employed when GnRHa is used to trigger ovulation (21). Otherwise, it will result in reduced implantation rates and increased miscarriage rates compared to hCG (22).

3.2.3 Dual Trigger

The "dual trigger" combines the benefits of the hCG and GnRHa to trigger ovulation. Theoretically, a low dose of hCG would be sufficient to avoid a suboptimal response to GnRHa trigger while maintaining a more effective luteal phase support without increasing the risk of OHSS (Figure 3.3) (23). In the last decades it has been used in distinct scenarios such as hyperresponders, poor response to COS, empty follicle syndrome or high proportion of immature oocytes in previous cycles, and also in normal responders (9, 24).

A recent systematic review showed that the dual trigger strategy is at least equivalent to GnRH or hCG alone in terms of number of oocytes retrieved, implantation rate and pregnancy rate in normal or hyperresponders (25). Unfortunately, reliable data on the

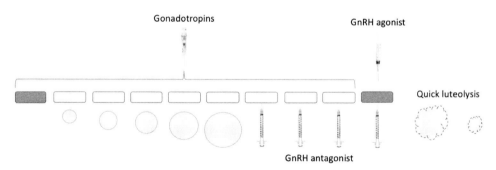

Figure 3.2 GnRHa trigger. Due to the quick luteolysis, additional drugs for luteal phase support are needed. A black and white version of this figure will appear in some formats. For the colour version, please refer to the plate section.

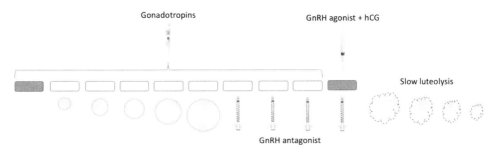

Figure 3.3 Dual trigger (GnRHa + hCG at the same time). Combines the advantage of reducing the risk of OHSS while maintaining an adequate luteal phase support and diminishing the incidence of EFS. A black and white version of this figure will appear in some formats. For the colour version, please refer to the plate section.

incidence of OHSS with the dual trigger strategy in hyperresponders is lacking, even though most studies reported reduced rates. Concerning the poor responders or those with a high proportion of immature oocytes in previous cycles, the dual trigger seems to ameliorate the number of oocytes obtained, implantation, and pregnancy rates (25). However, there is no consensus on the recommended dose of hCG in the dual trigger approach.

3.2.4 Double Trigger

The double trigger consists of the administration of GnRHa and hCG at 40 h and 34 h before oocyte pick-up, respectively (Figure 3.4) (26, 27). It has been suggested to improve the proportion of mature oocytes retrieved and to overcome some cases of empty follicle syndrome (EFS) (26, 28). Besides prolonging the interval between OT and oocyte retrieval, it offers the advantage of the hCG for luteal phase support. Nevertheless, there is insufficient data concerning the incidence of OHSS and premature ovulation with the double trigger.

A pilot study on granulosa cells gene expression showed that the double trigger strategy increased the expression of epiregulin and amphiregulin compared to hCG alone to trigger ovulation (29). A previous study demonstrated that the supplementation of the maturation medium with amphiregulin and epiregulin enhanced the maturation rate of human oocytes *in vitro* (30), which may explain the improved maturation, fertilization, and pregnancy rates among women that received the double trigger in that pilot study (29). Further basic studies may add important knowledge in the underlying mechanisms involved in human oocyte maturation.

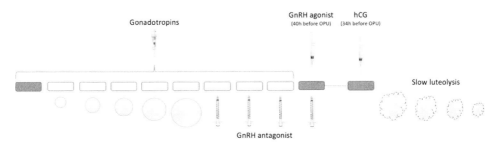

Figure 3.4 Double trigger (GnRHa at 40 hours before OPU + hCG at 34 hours before OPU). Follows the same principle as in the dual trigger strategy. A black and white version of this figure will appear in some formats. For the colour version, please refer to the plate section.

3.3 Suboptimal Response to GnRHa Trigger

The resumption of the meiosis in human oocytes occurs 14–18 hours after the onset of the LH surge (6), but the time interval since the onset of the LH surge and the threshold level of LH needed to induce follicular rupture are higher than those to induce oocyte maturation (31). Typically, LH levels greater than 15 IU/L continuing for 14–18 h is required for expanding cumulus cells that lead to ovulation trigger (32).

Low LH levels on the day of the OT is a risk factor for a suboptimal response to GnRHa. A recent study showed that LH levels inferior to 52 IU/L at 12 h after a bolus of GnRHa is suboptimal, while LH levels under 12 IU/L caused a dramatic reduction in oocyte yield and maturity (23). Serum LH levels greater than 15 IU/L at 12 h post-GnRHa trigger has been associated with significantly higher number of oocytes retrieved and increased oocyte maturity rate (23, 33). Furthermore, the lower the LH level after GnRHa trigger, the higher the suboptimal response rate (32). Indeed, LH levels inferior to 0.1 IU/L at the day of final oocyte maturation exhibit a suboptimal response rate nearly to 25 percent (32). However, regarding oocyte fertilization rate and clinical outcomes, a study failed to demonstrate statistically significance differences, as for the number of high-quality embryos and embryos transferred (33). An easier, cheaper and more convenient way to confirm that LH surge did happen after GnRHa trigger would be a urine LH test the morning after the trigger. We had shown that this is a very good alternative to blood sampling, avoiding patients coming again to the clinic, and with an excellent sensitivity (34).

Additional risk factors for suboptimal response to GnRHa trigger have been identified, such as very low basal FSH and LH levels at the start of stimulation and long-term hormonal contraception (32). Situations that lead to hypothalamic-pituitary axis suppression or dysfunction are believed to increase the risk of suboptimal response to GnRHa trigger, and the use of double trigger or dual trigger strategies may improve reproductive outcomes in these cases (32, 35).

In natural ovulatory cycles, the FSH preovulatory peak promotes the expression of LH receptors in granulosa cells and supports nuclear maturation along with cumulus development and expansion (4). Rosen et al. (36) reported significantly higher intrafollicular FSH concentration in follicles containing oocytes. Similarly, Lamb et al. (37), described a statistically significant improvement in oocyte recovery rate when concomitant FSH/hCG trigger injection was used compared to conventional hCG trigger alone. Nevertheless, whether an additional FSH bolus administered at the time of trigger enhances IVF outcomes requires further investigation.

3.4 Empty Follicle Syndrome

The empty follicle syndrome is a rare condition of uncertain etiology in which no oocytes are retrieved after technically correct oocyte pick-up (OPU) procedure, from apparently normally growing follicles during COS for assisted reproductive techniques (38). Although the exact etiology is not fully understood, a deficiency on loosening the cumulus oocyte complex from the follicles wall may play a role (38).

There are two types of EFS differentiated by the hormone levels on the day of OPU. The so-called genuine empty follicle syndrome happens when serum levels of hCG or LH are concordant with the correct administration of the triggering drug, while the false empty follicle syndrome (FEFS) occurs when such hormones levels are remarkably low (39).

The prevalence of EFS has been estimated to be around 2–7 percent (40). Most cases seem to be FEFS, which is commonly ascribed to a patient error in timing, preparation, or administration of the triggering drug, as well as to problems with manufacturing or shelf life (39). Abnormalities in the *in vivo* biological activity of some batches of commercially available hCG or GnRH and a rapid clearance of the hCG by the liver have also been described (41).

When problems in drug administration or quality were properly excluded, several hypotheses arise: early oocyte atresia due to a dysfunctional folliculogenesis in the presence of an apparently normal hormonal response; biological abnormality in oocyte supply despite normal bioavailability of hCG; and genetic factors such as LH/hCG receptor mutation or a blockage in the LH pathway (39, 40). Moreover, ovarian aging is considered a risk factor for EFS recurrence, probably due to altered folliculogenesis (42). In cases of GnRHa receptor polymorphism, higher doses of agonist are probably necessary in order to activate the receptor (39).

Finally, patients suffering from temporary or permanent hypothalamic-pituitary dysfunction should not receive GnRH agonist trigger, because a sufficient flare-up will not be achieved which will lead to a deficiency in follicular maturation and EFS (38). Borderline patients presenting with low circulating levels of both LH and FSH would also be at risk of developing EFS after GnRHa trigger (40).

3.5 Exaggerated Response to Ovulation Trigger

In different circumstances, some patients may have a hyperresponse to OT leading to OHSS, a life-threatening condition that occurs in the presence of prolonged LH activity, as seen after a hCG trigger. Such syndrome is characterized by an up regulation of vascular mediators that promote a sudden increase in capillary permeability culminating in rapid and massive fluid and electrolyte shift from the intravascular compartment to third space, which results in a massive enlargement of the ovaries and ascites (43).

Different vascular mediators released from the ovaries and other tissues in response to hCG have been described, such as vascular endothelial growth factor (VEGF), angiopoietin-2 (Ang-2), and vascular endothelial cadherin (44). VEGF is a cell-specific angiogenic and vasculogenic glycoprotein widely distributed in human tissues, especially at sites of angiogenesis. Its expression levels correlate with events requiring the growth of new blood vessels. In addition, VEGF plays roles in the induction of endothelial cell proliferation, migration, and micro vascular permeability (43).

Cerrillo et al. (44) hypothesized that GnRHa would induce a milder and shorter stimulus of vascular mediators involved in vascular leakage compared to hCG. Therefore, they studied the expression of VEGF, Ang-2, and VE-cadherin in egg donors that received either hCG or GnRHa to induce final oocyte maturation. Baseline characteristics and cycle parameters were similar between groups, but a shorter duration of the luteal phase was found in the group that received GnRHa. Likewise, abdominal pain or discomfort and bloating were significantly lower during the luteal phase on the GnRHa group. On the other hand, they did not find any difference in VEGF plasma levels between groups. However, there was a significant reduction in the VEGF concentration on follicular fluid from oocyte donors who received GnRHa. Similarly, VEGF mRNA expression was significantly lower in granulosa cells obtained from this group (44).

Currently, it is widely accepted that GnRHa trigger with subsequent elective frozen embryo transfer is the best strategy to avoid OHSS, avoiding both early OHHS due to exogenous hCG and late OHSS due to pregnancy-related endogenous hCG (9). Cases of severe OHSS after GnRHa trigger are almost anecdotal. Thus, patients at high risk of developing OHSS such as the hyperresponders should not be given hCG to trigger ovulation.

References

1. Sunkara SK, Rittenberg V, Raine-Fenning N, et al. Association between the number of eggs and live birth in IVF treatment: an analysis of 400 135 treatment cycles. Hum Reprod 2011;26:1768–1774.

2. Polyzos NP, Drakopoulos P, Parra J, et al. Cumulative live birth rates according to the number of oocytes retrieved after the first ovarian stimulation for in vitro fertilization/intracytoplasmic sperm injection: a multicenter multinational analysis including ~15,000 women. Fertil Steril 2018;110:661–670.

3. Conti M, Hsieh M, Musa Zamah A, et al. Novel signaling mechanisms in the ovary during oocyte maturation and ovulation. Mol Cell Endocrinol 2012;356:65–73.

4. Eppig JJ. FSH stimulates hyaluronic acid synthesis by oocyte-cumulus cell complexes from mouse preovulatory follicles. Nature 1979;281:483–484.

5. Andersen CY, Leonardsen L, Ulloa-Aguirre A, et al. FSH-induced resumption of meiosis in mouse oocytes: Effect of different isoforms. Mol Hum Reprod 1999;5:726–731.

6. Seibel MM, Smith DM, Levesque L, et al. The temporal relationship between the luteinizing hormone surge and human oocyte maturation. Am J Obstet Gynecol 1982;142:568–572.

7. Eppig JJ. Coordination of nuclear and cytoplasmic oocyte maturation in eutherian mammals. In: *Reproduction, Fertility and Development*. CSIRO, 1996:485–489.

8. Scott RT, Hofmann GE, Muasher SJ, et al. Correlation of follicular diameter with oocyte recovery and maturity at the time of transvaginal follicular aspiration. J Vitr Fertil Embryo Transf 1989;6:73–75.

9. Dosouto C, Haahr T, Humaidan P. Advances in ovulation trigger strategies. Panminerva Med 2019;61:42–51.

10. Castillo JC, Humaidan P, Bernabéu R. Pharmaceutical options for triggering of final oocyte maturation in ART. BioMed Res Int 2014. doi:10.1155/2014/580171. [Epub ahead of print]

11. Loumaye E, Engrand P, Arguinzoniz M, et al. Recombinant human luteinizing hormone is as effective as, but safer than, urinary human chorionic gonadotropin in inducing final follicular maturation and ovulation in in vitro fertilization procedures: Results of a multicenter double-blind study. J Clin Endocrinol Metab 2001;86:2607–2618.

12. Casarini L, Santi D, Brigante G, et al. Two hormones for one receptor: evolution, biochemistry, actions, and pathophysiology of LH and hCG. Endocrine Rev 2018;39:549–592.

13. Huhtaniemi IT, Catt KJ. Differential binding affinities of rat testis luteinizing hormone (lH) receptors for human chorionic gonadotropin, human lH, and ovine LH. Endocrinology 1981;108:1931–1938.

14. Huhtaniemi IT, Clayton RN, Catt KJ. Gonadotropin binding and leydig cell activation in the rat testis in vivo. Endocrinology 1982;111:982–987.

15. Youssef MA, Abou-Setta AM, Lam WS. Recombinant versus urinary human chorionic gonadotrophin for final oocyte maturation triggering in IVF and ICSI cycles. Cochrane Database Syst Rev 2016. doi:10.1002/14651858.CD003719.pub4. [Epub ahead of print]

16. Gonen Y, Balakier H, Powell W, et al. Use of gonadotropin-releasing hormone agonist to trigger follicular maturation for in vitro fertilization. J Clin Endocrinol Metab 1990;71:918–922.

17. Dosouto C, Haahr T, Humaidan P. Gonadotropin-releasing hormone agonist (GnRHa) trigger – state of the art. Reprod Biol 2017;17:1–8.

18. Itskovitz J, Boldes R, Levron J, et al. Induction of preovulatory luteinizing hormone surge and prevention of ovarian hyperstimulation syndrome by gonadotropin-releasing hormone agonist. Fertil Steril 1991;56:213–220.

19. Griesinger G, Diedrich K, Devroey P, et al. GnRH agonist for triggering final oocyte maturation in the GnRH antagonist ovarian hyperstimulation protocol: a systematic review and meta-analysis. Hum Reprod Update 2006;12:159–168.

20. Kolibianakis EM, Schultze-Mosgau A, Schroer A, et al. A lower ongoing pregnancy rate can be expected when GnRH agonist is used for triggering final oocyte maturation instead of HCG in patients undergoing IVF with GnRH antagonists. Hum Reprod 2005;20:2887–2892.

21. Haahr T, Roque M, Esteves SC, et al. GnRH agonist trigger and LH activity luteal phase support versus hcg trigger and conventional luteal phase support in fresh embryo transfer IVF/ICSI cycles-a systematic PRISMA review and meta-analysis. Front Endocrinol 2017;8. doi:10.3389/fendo.2017.00116. [Epub ahead of print]

22. Youssef MAFM, Van der Veen F, Al-Inany HG, et al. Gonadotropin-releasing hormone agonist versus HCG for oocyte triggering in antagonist-assisted reproductive technology. Cochrane Database Syst Rev 2014. doi:10.1002/14651858.CD008046.pub4. [Epub ahead of print]

23. Shapiro BS, Daneshmand ST, Restrepo H, et al. Efficacy of induced luteinizing hormone surge after "trigger" with gonadotropin-releasing hormone agonist. Fertil Steril 2011;95:826–828.

24. Fabris AM, Cruz M, Legidos V, et al. Dual triggering with gonadotropin-releasing hormone agonist and standard dose human chorionic gonadotropin in patients with a high immature oocyte rate. Reprod Sci 2017;24:1221–1225.

25. De Oliveira SA, Calsavara VF, Cortés GC. Final oocyte maturation in assisted reproduction with human chorionic gonadotropin and gonadotropin-releasing hormone agonist (dual trigger). J Bras Reprod Assist 2016;20:246–250.

26. Haas J, Zilberberg E, Dar S, et al. Co-administration of GnRH agonist and hCG for final oocyte maturation (double trigger) in patients with low number of oocytes retrieved per number of preovulatory follicles-a preliminary report. J Ovarian Res 2014;7. doi:10.1186/1757-2215-7-77. [Epub ahead of print]

27. Orvieto R. Triggering final follicular maturation-hCG, GnRH agonist or both, when and to whom? J Ovarian Res 2015;8:60.

28. Beck-Fruchter R, Weiss A, Lavee M, et al. Empty follicle syndrome: successful treatment in a recurrent case and review of the literature. Hum Reprod 2012;27:1357–1367.

29. Haas J, Ophir L, Barzilay E, et al. Standard human chorionic gonadotropin versus double trigger for final oocyte maturation results in different granulosa cells gene expressions: a pilot study. Fertil Steril 2016;106:653–659.

30. Ben-Ami I, Komsky A, Bern O, et al. In vitro maturation of human germinal vesicle-stage oocytes: role of epidermal growth factor-like growth factors in the culture medium. Hum Reprod 2011;26:76–81.

31. Peluso JJ. Role of the amplitude of the gonadotropin surge in the rat. Fertil Steril 1990;53:150–154.

32. Meyer L, Murphy LA, Gumer A, et al. Risk factors for a suboptimal response to gonadotropin-releasing hormone agonist trigger during in vitro fertilization cycles. Fertil Steril 2015;104:637–642.

33. Chen SL, Ye DS, Chen X, et al. Circulating luteinizing hormone level after triggering oocyte maturation with GnRH agonist may predict oocyte yield in flexible GnRH antagonist protocol. Hum Reprod 2012;27:1351–1356.

34. Cozzolino M, Matey S, Alvarez A, Toribio M, López V, Perona M, Henzenn E, Piró M, Humaidan P, Garcia-Velasco JA. Self-detection of the LH surge in urine after

GnRH agonist trigger in IVF – how to minimize failure to retrieve oocytes. Front Endocrinol 2020;11:221.

35. Lu X, Hong Q, Sun LH, et al. Dual trigger for final oocyte maturation improves the oocyte retrieval rate of suboptimal responders to gonadotropin-releasing hormone agonist. Fertil Steril 2016;106:1356–1362.

36. Rosen MP, Zamah AM, Shen S, et al. The effect of follicular fluid hormones on oocyte recovery after ovarian stimulation: FSH level predicts oocyte recovery. Reprod Biol Endocrinol 2009;7. doi:10.1186/1477-7827-7-35. [Epub ahead of print]

37. Lamb JD, Shen S, McCulloch C, et al. Follicle-stimulating hormone administered at the time of human chorionic gonadotropin trigger improves oocyte developmental competence in in vitro fertilization cycles: a randomized, double-blind, placebo-controlled trial. Fertil Steril 2011;95:1655–1660.

38. Castillo JC, García-Velasco J, Humaidan P. Empty follicle syndrome after GnRHa triggering versus hCG triggering in COS. J Assist Reprod Genet 2012;29:249–253.

39. Blazquez A, Guillén JJ, Colomé C, et al. Empty follicle syndrome prevalence and management in oocyte donors. Hum Reprod 2014;29:2221–2227.

40. Ben-Shlomo I, Schiff E, Levran D, et al. Failure of oocyte retrieval during in vitro fertilization: a sporadic event rather than a syndrome. Fertil Steril 1991;55:324–327.

41. Zegers-Hochschild F, Fernández E, Mackenna A, et al. The empty follicle syndrome: a pharmaceutical industry syndrome. Hum Reprod 1995;10:2262–2265.

42. Zreik TG, García-Velasco J, Vergara T, et al. Empty follicle syndrome: evidence for recurrence. Hum Reprod 2000;15:999–1002.

43. Ajonuma LC. Is vascular endothelial growth factor (VEGF) the main mediator in ovarian hyperstimulation syndrome (OHSS)? Med Hypotheses 2008;70:1174–1178.

44. Cerrillo M, Pacheco A, Rodríguez S, et al. Effect of GnRH agonist and hCG treatment on VEGF, angiopoietin-2, and VE-cadherin: trying to explain the link to ovarian hyperstimulation syndrome. Fertil Steril 2011;95:2517–2519.

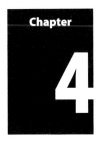

Individualized Luteal Phase Support

Barbara Lawrenz and Human M. Fatemi

4.1 Introduction

In ovarian stimulation cycles for IVF/ICSI, a defective luteal phase occurs in almost all patients as a result of the multifollicular development and supraphysiological hormonal levels, which inhibit the LH secretion by the pituitary via negative feedback actions at the level of the hypothalamic-pituitary axis. Progesterone is crucial to induce secretory transformation of the endometrium after previous estrogenization, a process which will finally result in a receptive endometrium. Consequently, luteal phase support (LPS) represents an essential part of ART treatment in case of a planned fresh embryo transfer, as it is crucial to counterbalance the luteal phase insufficiency.

The endocrine profile of the luteal phase is influenced substantially from the medication, used for final oocyte maturation. Depending on the stimulation protocol and the ovarian response of the patient, either hCG, a GnRH agonist, or the combination of both are used for final oocyte maturation. The task of the reproductive medicine specialist is to tailor the LPS according to the patient´s specific characteristics and the stimulation protocol. Therefore this chapter aims to describe the physiology of the luteal phase in the natural cycle, the different endocrine profiles in the luteal phase of ovarian stimulation cycles, the existing approaches for LPS and the necessity, as well as the possibilities, to individualize LPS.

4.2 Physiology of the Luteal Phase in a Natural Cycle

The luteal phase of a menstrual cycle is the time between ovulation and, in case of conception, the establishment of a pregnancy or otherwise the onset of menses.

In a natural cycle, estradiol synthesis increases progressively from the dominant follicle and initiates LH surge. Even before the LH surge, a small increase in progesterone levels is seen, which reflects the increasing LH pulse amplitude and frequency leading up to the surge. A LH surge of 24–36 hours is sufficient to initiate the resumption of oocyte meiosis, luteinization of granulosa cells, ovulation, and the initial phase of corpora lutea development. Progesterone and 17α-hydroxyprogesterone (17α-OHP) plasma concentrations increase rapidly after the LH surge, indicating the beginning of granulosa and theca cell luteinization. The hormonal activity of the corpus luteum depends on the pulsatile LH secretion resulting in a production of up to 40 mg of progesterone per day and additional a significant amount of androgens and estradiol. LH pulses during the luteal phase are of a reduced frequency and of a greater amplitude than in the follicular phase and during the course of the luteal phase, the mean LH pulse frequency declines from 15.2 pulses/24 h in the early to 8.4/24 h in the late luteal phase (1). Also a reduction in the amplitude of LH pulses was also observed in the late luteal phase.

In case of a conception, the embryo will start to produce human chorionic gonadotropin (hCG) from day 7 of fertilization. hCG has structural similarities with LH and activates the same receptor. Therefore the hCG, produced by the embryo, will counterbalance the subsiding LH pulses and maintain the hormonal activity of the corpus luteum until the progesterone production shifts from the corpus luteum to the placenta at around 9 weeks of pregnancy. Without a conception, luteolysis will occur as a physiological process of corpus luteum regression. Functional luteolysis with reduced secretion of progesterone is followed by structural luteolysis.

4.3 Physiology of the Luteal Phase in Ovarian Stimulation Cycles for IVF/ICSI

In stimulated cycles for IVF, a defective luteal phase occurs in almost all patients (2). Initially it was thought that the defective luteal phase was due to the aspiration of a large number of granulosa cells during oocyte retrieval procedure. Later on it was demonstrated that the reason for the luteal phase insufficiency, seen after controlled ovarian stimulation, seems to be the multifollicular development achieved during the follicular phase. In IVF/ICSI treatment daily dosages of exogenous gonadotropins are administered to support multifollicular growth with the aim of maximizing the number of available oocytes for fertilization, resulting in a large number of growing follicles and supraphysiological hormonal levels. These supraphysiological levels inhibit the LH secretion by the pituitary via negative feedback actions at the level of the hypothalamic-pituitary axis (3).

Final oocyte maturation is the crucial step in ovarian stimulation cycles for IVF in order to retrieve mature oocytes for further processing in the IVF laboratory. Whereas in GnRH (Gonadotropin-releasing-hormone)-agonist cycles, only hCG can be administered for final oocyte maturation, in GnRH antagonist cycles, hCG as well as GnRH-agonists can be used. However, due to the different ways of action of hCG and GnRH agonist, the endocrine profile of the luteal phase in stimulated cycles depends substantially from the medication used for final oocyte maturation.

Table 4.1 summarizes the differences between the natural and the stimulated cycle.

4.4 Endocrine Profile of the Luteal Phase after HCG Trigger

As described above, under physiological conditions ovulation is induced by a rise in LH levels. In the early years of IVF treatment, purified LH was not commercially available at adequate doses to support final follicular maturation, therefore hCG was used instead routinely for final oocyte maturation. HCG is a glycoprotein hormone with the typical heterodimeric structure also exhibited by LH, FSH, and TSH. These hormones share a common α-subunit but have distinctly different ß-subunits. hCG and LH have 85 percent of the amino acid sequence of their ß-subunit in common. The main differences between them lie within the N-linked oligosaccharides and the C-terminal sequence. The latter, and especially the O-linked oligosaccharides in this peptide, are responsible for the longer half-life of hCG compared with LH. Nowadays hCG is available in urinary and recombinant form, both with a comparable half-life time of approximately 30 hours (4). HCG attaches to and activates the same receptor as LH and is therefore capable to induce final oocyte maturation. The most important difference between LH and hCG is the difference in half-life, which is 6–8 times longer for hCG compared to LH. The longer half-life of hCG is the

Table 4.1 Endocrine profile of the luteal phase in natural cycles and ovarian stimulation cycles

	Natural cycle	**Ovarian stimulation cycle**	
Ovulation	Induced by LH surge	Final oocyte maturation with hCG or dual trigger	Final oocyte maturation with GnRH agonist
Early luteal phase	Pulsatile LH secretion will maintain the progesterone production by the corpus lutem	Progesterone production stimulated by hCG, activating LH receptor, duration max 5 days	Progesterone production stimulated by LH, resulting from flare-up, duration approx. 2 days. Supraphysiological levels inhibit the LH secretion via negative feedback, leading to luteolysis
Late luteal phase	*No conception:* subsiding LH pulses will lead to Corpus luteum regression and luteolysis *Conception:* hCG from the embryo will activate the LH receptor	Supraphysiological levels inhibit the LH secretion via negative feedback, leading to luteolysis of different extent	Mostly characterized by severe luteolysis

crucial factor for the higher risk of ovarian hyperstimulation syndrome (OHSS), especially in the high-responder patient. When the hCG stimulus on the corpora lutea subsides, luteolysis will occur due to a lack of endogenous LH.

4.5 Endocrine Profile of the Luteal Phase after GnRH Agonist Trigger

Contrary to hCG, the GnRH-agonist acts by dislocating the GnRH antagonist from the GnRH receptors in the pituitary and its administration results in a surge of LH and FSH (so-called flare-up). This surge is sufficient to induce final oocyte maturation and ovulation (5). Despite the fact that the application of a GnRH agonist trigger in a GnRH antagonist protocol imitates the natural mid-cycle surge of LH and FSH and the magnitude of natural and GnRH agonist–induced LH surges are comparable, distinct differences between both are found. The spontaneous LH surge in a natural cycle is characterized by an ascending phase of approximately 4 hours, a peak plateau of 20 hours, and a descending phase of 20 hours whereas the GnRHa-induced LH/FSH surge has a significantly shorter ascending phase. The differences between natural and artificial induced LH surge cannot be overcome by an increase in the GnRH agonist dosage or by repeat GnRH agonist administration. As the duration of the LH/FSH surge is critical for a normal luteal function and an LH increment of too short a duration prevents the granulosa cells from completing luteinization, further on impairs the secretory function of the corpus luteum is commonly impaired and the life-span is shortened. At the same time, the supraphysiological levels of estradiol and progesterone after ovarian stimulation alter LH secretion from the pituitary via negative feedback mechanisms. Pulsatile LH secretion from the pituitary continues, however the mean LH concentration and LH pulse amplitude are lower compared to the natural cycle. Hence, the process of luteolysis starts very early in the luteal phase which is demonstrated by the decline of progesterone and estradiol levels two days after ovulation (6). Previously it was believed that the luteal phase is always characterized by severe luteolysis and luteal phase insufficiency as a result of the short duration of the induced LH/FSH peak after GnRH agonist administration (7). Interestingly, luteolysis after GnRH-agonist trigger is not always complete and may vary, indicating individual differences among patients. It seems that longer stimulation duration as well as a higher level of progesterone on the day of final oocyte maturation and more retrieved oocytes will result in higher levels of progesterone 48 hours after oocyte retrieval, pointing toward a sustained secretory capability of the corpora lutea even after GnRHa trigger (8).

In patients, considered to be at risk for OHSS development, final oocyte maturation by administration of a GnRH agonist in a GnRH antagonist protocol is meanwhile considered as the "gold standard" as it leads to a significant reduction in the incidence of OHSS (9). Hence it has to be noted, that even GnRH agonist trigger does not completely avoided development of OHSS. Table 4.2 presents the different approaches for final oocyte maturation and their implications for the luteal phase.

4.6 Progesterone and Endometrial Receptivity

Progesterone induces the secretory transformation of the endometrium after previous estrogenization, a process which is dependent from the time of progesterone exposure and which will finally result in a receptive endometrium.

Endometrial receptivity, a good quality, euploid embryo at blastocyst developmental stage and the synchrony between both are mandatory for successful implantation (10). The implantation process is characterized by the apposition of a blastocyst-stage embryo to a receptive endometrium, the attachment to the maternal endometrial epithelium and finally the invasion into the endometrial stroma. It is well known that an embryo has the ability to implant in different tissues outside the uterine cavity, nevertheless, implantation in the endometrium can only occur when the endometrium is receptive. This phase is nowadays referred to as the "window of implantation" (WOI). It is interesting to note that this nowadays well recognized and often used phrase was first described long before the first successful IVF treatment (11).

Due to ethical considerations, the exact duration of the WOI is difficult to define in humans. In an idealized 28 day cycle, it is assumed that the WOI takes place between day 19 and day 21 of the menstrual cycle, however different durations are described, from 48 hours up to possibly 4 days (12, 13). The methods taken to identify endometrial receptivity in the human endometrium have changed over the last decades. Changes of the endometrium, occurring under the influence of progesterone, have been described histologically already in 1950. Later on, it was demonstrated that the endometrium at the time of receptivity expresses proteins, thought to facilitate and promote implantation and a family of cell surface glycoproteins, so-called integrins, were identified. Their expression in the endometrium appeared to be cyclical during the menstrual cycle and particularly "up-regulated" during the WOI. Currently endometrial receptivity is investigated by gene expression patterns (14).

Table 4.2 Characteristics of the type of final oocyte maturation and implications for the luteal phase

	hCG	GnRH-agonist
Mode of action	Activation of the LH receptor	dislocates the GnRH antagonist from the GnRH receptors in the pituitary and results in a LH/FSH surge of LH and FSH
Implication for luteal phase	Risk for OHSS development due to half-life of approximately 30 hours	Risk for severe luteolysis

4.7 Luteal Phase Support in ART Cycles

To counterbalance the luteal phase insufficiency after ovarian stimulation and to maintain the secretory endometrium, an adequate luteal phase support is crucial and a must after ovarian stimulation in case of a planned fresh embryo transfer.

In a natural cycle, luteal phase deficiency (LPD) was defined as having mid-luteal progesterone levels below 10 ng/mL (31.8 nmol/L) or a sum of three random serum P measurements < 30 ng/mL (95.4 nmol/L) (15). The correction of a dysfunctional corpus luteum with the symptoms shortened luteal phase and premenstrual spotting, by adminis-tration of progesterone, was first described in 1949 (16) and a defective luteal phase was defined, if the serum mid-luteal progesterone levels are less than 10 ng/mL. Prevalence of luteal phase defect (LPD) in natural cycles in normo-ovulatory patients with primary or secondary infertility was demonstrated to be about 8.1 percent. However in 2012, the ASRM stated that there is no reproducible, physiologically relevant, and clinically practical stan-dard to diagnose LPD or distinguish fertile from infertile women (17). The minimum threshold of progesterone level that is essential for the maintenance of a pregnancy is unknown and successful pregnancies have been reported even when the concentration of progesterone was never above 15 nmol/L for the first 14 days.

In IVF treatments, the lower limit of progesterone levels to achieve and maintain a pregnancy is not defined yet. It seems that a progesterone level of more than 30 ng/mL and an estradiol level of more than 100 pg/mL at the day of implantation are more likely to have a viable and ongoing pregnancy compared to patients with hormone levels below these thresholds. Other publications report successful pregnancies with mid-luteal progesterone levels above 17 ng/mL or even as low as a progesterone level above 15 ng/mL two days after GnRH-agonist trigger, provided that adequate luteal phase support was applied.

In the last years, there is an increasing trend to tailor treatment approach according to the patient´s characteristics as a consequence of the increasing knowledge on interpatient variability. This knowledge challenges the old concept of one type of luteal phase support for all IVF patients and advocate to implement a personalized approach into daily clinical routine, which depends on the type of final oocyte maturation and the ovarian response.

4.8 Strategies for Luteal Phase Support

Vaginal progesterone administration is worldwide the preferred route of LPS. Maximal serum levels of progesterone are reached three to eight hours after application of vaginal suppositories or tablets, and thereafter, they fall continuously over the next eight hours.

Sufficient luteal phase plasma levels are achieved by daily administration of 300 – 600 mg of progesterone, divided into 2 or 3 dosages (18) and the vaginal absorption is influenced by the kind of formula preparation and is enhanced after previous estrogenization. Despite the fact, that serum progesterone levels when measured using vaginal progesterone administration are sometimes even lower than in a natural cycle, adequate secretory endometrial transformation is achieved. Obviously, the vaginally administered progesterone exerts a direct local effect on the endometrium before it enters the systemic circulation. This is described as the "first uterine pass"-effect; hence the underlying mechanism of which is not fully understood. Possible side effects of the vaginal progesterone administration are increased vaginal discharge and possible vaginal irritation. In case of severe side effects with vaginal use, patients can be advised to administer progesterone rectally.

Oral administration would offer a convenient way of progesterone administration. Since natural progesterone is rapidly metabolized after oral intake, it is ineffective in inducing a sufficient secretory transformation and the side effects of synthetic progesterone derivatives on lipids and on the psyche limit their use. Through the process of micronization of progesterone the absorption and bioavailability have been improved, hence even higher doses of micronized progesterone have failed to induce sufficient secretory transformation. Recently, some data have confirmed the efficacy of a daily intake of 30 mg dydrogesterone as luteal phase support. If confirmed in larger studies, oral progesterone may be a more easy and convenient way of progesterone administration (19).

Intramuscular progesterone administration is accompanied by several disadvantages: the need of daily i.m. injections, the pain experienced by the patient at injection time, the possible swelling and redness and also the possible danger of a sterile abscess formation. A rare but more severe and even life-threatening complication is the development of eosinophilic pneumonia after progesterone i.m. injections for luteal phase support as an allergic reaction toward the oil vehicle, used as excipient for the substance itself. Progesterone is rapidly absorbed after i.m. injection and high progesterone plasma concentrations are reached after approximately two hours with peak concentrations around eight hours after injection. A daily dosage of 25 mg progesterone is required to achieve progesterone levels, which are equivalent to those of the luteal phase in a natural cycle. It seems, that the intramuscular injection site serves as a progesterone depot and sustains serum concentration of progesterone. Subcutaneous progesterone injections could pose an alternative for women, who want to avoid i.m. injections as well as the vaginal route. As no superiority of one administration route over the other has been shown to have an impact on ART outcome, also the patients´ preference can be considered when choosing the route of progesterone administration for luteal phase support.

The concept of hCG administration as luteal phase support mimics the physiology of corpus luteum maintenance by an implanting and developing embryo. For a long time, hCG was considered to be the gold standard for LPS. Through the application of hCG, the corpora lutea will be stimulated continuously and will therefore sustain progesterone production. The risk of hCG administrations as a means of LPS is the possible development of ovarian hyperstimulation syndrome (OHSS), which may affect especially the patients with a good ovarian reserve and response to ovarian stimulation. Some data even point to a possible interference of the hCG, administered for LPS, and the hyperglycosylated hCG (H-hCG), secreted by the developing embryo and to which an important role in implantation is contributed (20). Table 4.3 summarizes the available strategies for LPS

Table 4.3 Strategies for LPS

	hCG	Progesterone		
Way of administration	Subcutaneous	Vaginal/rectal	i.m.	Oral (Dydrogesterone)
Advantages	Can be performed without any additional exogenous progesterone	No injections needed		Patient-friendly approach
Risks/side effects	Possible OHSS development	– Vaginal discharge – As sole LPS not sufficient after GnRH-agonist trigger	– Painful injection – Sterile abscess formation – Need of assistance for administration	Further data for final confirmation warranted
Dosages	– 125 IU daily – 2,500 IU 2× during luteal phase – 375–1500 IU as single bolus, depending on progesterone level	– 300–600 mg, depending on formula used	– 25 mg daily after hCG trigger – 50 mg daily after GnRH-agonist trigger	– 30 mg daily

4.9 Luteal Phase Support after Induction of Final Oocyte Maturation with HCG

HCG and LH activate the same receptor and besides the capability of hCG to induce final oocyte maturation, hCG maintains corpora lutea function in the early luteal phase for up to five days due to its half-life time of more than 24 hours.

After hCG administration for final oocyte maturation, LPS can be performed either with hCG alone, progesterone alone, or the combination of both. Repeatedly applied hCG in a dosage up to 2.500 IU, is known to be efficient in sustaining corpora lutea function, however, this approach is accompanied by the risk of OHSS development. Also no significant favorable effect of progesterone in combination with hCG compared to exogenous progesterone alone was found in a Cochrane analysis (21).

Based on the experience with low-dose hCG administration for LPS after GnRH-agonist trigger, a mathematical model was designed to calculate the daily applied hCG dosage, required to maintain sufficient hCG concentrations (20). Preliminary results indicate, that 100 IU hCG, daily applied, seems to be sufficient even without any additional exogenous progesterone, to maintain the corpora lutea function until endogenous hCG from the developing embryo takes over. Unfortunately, the aforementioned small dosages of hCG are not commercially available rendering it difficult to implement this as a clinical routine.

4.10 Luteal Phase Support after Final Oocyte Maturation with GnRH Agonist

As described above, the GnRH agonist–induced LH flare is remarkably shorter as compared to the natural LH surge, leading in most patients to an early luteolysis and luteal phase insufficiency. The first studies which used GnRH agonist for final oocyte maturation, showed significantly lower pregnancy rates (22), caused by the luteal phase insufficiency. Besides an aggressive LPS with estradiol administration and daily applied doses of 50 mg i.m. progesterone, severe luteolysis can also be counterbalanced by hCG, to be given not later than 72 hours after GnRH agonist trigger. Rescue of the corpora lutea can be performed up to 3 days of gonadotropin deprivation and is hCG dose dependent, requiring a minimum dose of 1500 IU hCG and more. Following this concept, it was shown that GnRH-agonist triggering, followed by 1.500 IU hCG given 35 hours later, resulted in the same pregnancy rates as compared to a 10.000 IU hCG trigger. Alternatively daily low-dose hCG in dosages of 125 IU rec-hCG are also sufficient to sustain progesterone levels, even without the use of exogenous progesterone. However, both approaches may still lead to OHSS in high-responder patients.

As some patients will not be affected by luteolysis, the crucial step is to identify these patients. By individualizing their LPS, "overtreatment" can be avoided. The concept of "luteal coasting" is based on the patient´s specific luteolysis pattern by applying individualized hCG doses, according to the progesterone levels measured in the early and mid-luteal phase (23). Depending on the progesterone level 48 hours post-oocyte retrieval, a single hCG dosage between 375 and 1.500 IU, given in early luteal phase, can maintain adequate progesterone levels and this approach may well optimize the chance of pregnancy while reducing the risk of OHSS associated with higher doses of hCG supplementation in the luteal phase (24). The necessity for repeat blood tests to measure progesterone levels poses the most important

Table 4.4 Possibilities for LPS, depending on the medication used for final oocyte maturation

	Medication used for final oocyte maturation	
	hCG	GnRH agonist
Possibilities of luteal phase support	– vaginal progesterone – i.m. progesterone – hCG – oral dydrogesterone (more data required)	– i.m. progesterone and estradiol – hCG – "luteal coasting" (hCG dosage according to progesterone level)

disadvantage of this approach. In case of implantation, endogenously produced hCG from the embryo will compensate for the LH deficit and avoid regression of the corpora lutea. The possibilities of different approaches for LPS, depending on the medications used for final oocyte maturation, are summarized in Table 4.4.

4.11 Timing of Luteal Phase Support with Progesterone

Timing of luteal phase support start is crucial, as it has to be initiated before endogenous progesterone levels are decreasing or are too low. Hence, preovulatory exposure of the endometrium to progesterone may have a negative impact on the endometrial receptivity and start of progesterone administration before oocyte retrieval procedure was found to decrease the likelihood of pregnancy, when compared to start on the day of oocyte retrieval. There is no difference in the clinical pregnancy rate when progesterone is initiated on the evening of oocyte retrieval versus start on day 1–3 after oocyte retrieval. However, when progesterone administration was started on day 6, a decreased likelihood of pregnancy was found. Therefore, initiation of progesterone supplementation between the evening of oocyte retrieval and day 3 after retrieval seems to be ideal (25).

4.12 Duration of the Luteal Phase Support

In early pregnancy, rapidly increasing amounts of hCG are produced by the embryo. This embryo derived hCG will replace a possible lack of endogenous LH after ovarian stimulation until the progesterone production has shifted from the corpora lutea toward the placenta. Studies evaluating the duration of progesterone administration after a positive pregnancy test did not find any influence on the miscarriage rate and the delivery rate when progesterone application was continued or discontinued for 3 weeks after positive pregnancy test (26).

4.13 Conclusion

Estradiol and progesterone are essential for human reproduction to prepare the endometrium for implantation. In ovarian stimulation cycles for IVF/ICSI, multifollicular follicle growth with supraphysiological hormonal levels will inhibit LH secretion from the pituitary via negative feedback actions. As a consequence, the luteal phase of these ovarian stimulation cycles are mostly characterized by severe luteal phase insufficiency and adequate LPS is a must in cycles, when a fresh embryo transfer is planned.

In recent years, ovarian stimulation is increasingly tailored according to the patient´s characteristics, hence LPS is still often performed in a "one-size-fits-all" approach. In future, reproductive medicine specialists need to individualize LPS not only to the patient´s specific needs and desires, but also to the type of treatment performed. The greatest indication for individualization of the luteal phase is required in high-responder patients, following GnRH-agonist trigger, in order to tailor the LPS to the patient-specific pattern of luteolysis and minimize the risk of OHSS.

References

1. Filicori M, Santoro N, Merriam GR, et al. Characterization of the physiological pattern of episodic gonadotropin secretion throughout the human menstrual cycle. J Clin Endocrinol Metab 1986;62:1136–1144.

2. Kolibianakis EM, Devroey P. The luteal phase after ovarian stimulation. Reprod Biomed Online 2002a;5:26–35.

3. Fatemi HM. The luteal phase after 3 decades of IVF: what do we know? Reprod Biomed Online 2009;19(Suppl 4):4331.

4. Ludwig M, Doody KJ, Doody KM. Use of recombinant human chorionic gonadotropin in ovulation induction. Fertil Steril 2003;79(5):1051–1059.

5. Gonen Y, Balakier H, Powell W, et al. Use of gonadotropin-releasing hormone agonist to trigger follicular maturation for in vitro fertilization. J Clin Endocrinol Metab 1990;71:918–922.

6. Tannus S, Burke Y, McCartney CR, et al. GnRH-agonist triggering for final oocyte maturation in GnRH-antagonist IVF cycles induces decreased LH pulse rate and amplitude in early luteal phase: a possible luteolysis mechanism. Gynecol Endocrinol 2017. [Epub ahead of print]

7. Fatemi HM, Polyzos NP, van Vaerenbergh I, et al. Early luteal phase endocrine profile is affected by the mode of triggering final oocyte maturation and the luteal phase support used in recombinant follicle-stimulating hormone–gonadotropin-releasing hormone antagonist in vitro fertilization cycles. Fertil Steril 2013;100:742–747.

8. Lawrenz B, Garrido N, Samir S, et al. Individual luteolysis pattern after GnRH-agonist trigger for final oocyte maturation. PLoS One 2017;12(5): e0176600.

9. Devroey P, Polyzos NP, Blockeel C. An OHSS-free clinic by segmentation of IVF treatment. Hum Reprod 2011;26:2593–2597.

10. Simon C, Martin JC, Pellicer A. Paracrine regulators of implantation. Baillieres Best Pract Res Clin Obstet Gynaecol 2000;14:815–826.

11. Psychoyos A. Hormonal control of ovoimplantation. Vitam Horm 1973;31:201–256.

12. Giudice LC. Genes associated with embryonic attachment and implantation and the role of progesterone. J Reprod Med 1999;44:165–171.

13. Kodaman P, Taylor H. Hormonal regulation of implantation. Obstet Gynecol Clin N Am 2004;31:745–766.

14. Díaz-Gimeno P, Horcajadas JA, Martínez-Conejero JA, et al. A genomic diagnostic tool for human endometrial receptivity based on the transcriptomic signature. Fertil Steril 2011;95(1):50–60.

15. Jordan J, Craig K, Clifton DK, et al. Luteal phase defect: the sensitivity and specificity of diagnostic methods in common clinical use. Fertil Steril 1994;62(1):54–62.

16. Jones GES. Some new aspects of management of infertility. JAMA 1979;141:1123.

17. Practice Committee of the American Society for Reproductive Medicine. Current clinical irrelevance of luteal phase deficiency: a committee opinion. Fertil Steril 2015;103:e27–33.

18. Devroey P, Palermo G, Bourgain C, et al. Progesterone administration in patients

with absent ovaries. Int J Fertil 1989;34:188–193.

19. Griesinger G, Blockeel C, Tournaye H. Oral dydrogesterone for luteal phase support in fresh in vitro fertilization cycles: a new standard? Fertil Steril 2018;109 (5):756–762.

20. Andersen CY, Fischer R, Giorgione V, et al. Micro-dose hCG as luteal phase support without exogenous progesterone administration: mathematical modelling of the hCG concentration in circulation and initial clinical experience. J Assist Reprod Genet 2016;33(10):1311–1318.

21. van der Linden M, Buckingham K, Farquhar C, et al. Luteal phase support for assisted reproduction cycles. Cochrane Database Syst Rev 2015;7(7):CD009154.

22. Humaidan P, Bredkjaer HE, Bungum L, et al. GnRH agonist (buserelin) or hCG for ovulation induction in GnRH antagonist IVF/ICSI cycles: a prospective randomized study. Hum Reprod 2005;20:1213–1220.

23. Kol S, Breyzman T, Segal L, et al. "Luteal coasting" after GnRH agonist trigger – individualized, HCG-based, progesterone-free luteal support in "high responders": a case series. RBMonline 2015;31:747–751.

24. Lawrenz B, Samir S, Garrido N, et al. Luteal coasting and individualization of human chorionic gonadotropin dose after gonadotropin-releasing hormone agonist triggering for final oocyte maturation – a retrospective proof-of-concept study. Front Endocrinol (Lausanne) 2018;15(9):33.

25. Connell MT, Szatkowski JM, Terry N, et al. Timing luteal support in assisted reproductive technology: a systematic review. Fertil Steril 2015;103:939–946.

26. Nyboe AA, Popovic-Todorovic B, Schmidt KT, et al. Progesterone supplementation during early gestations after IVF or ICSI has no effect on the delivery rates: a randomized controlled trial. Hum Reprod 2002;17:357–361.

Chapter 5

Individualized Management of Male Infertility

Matheus Roque

5.1 Introduction

Approximately 8–15 percent of couples are unable to conceive after one year of unprotected intercourse, and they are thereby considered infertile; this problem has become a global health concern, affecting roughly 187 million couples worldwide (1). Male factor infertility occurs in 40–50 percent of the infertile couples, being solely responsible in approximately 20 percent of cases and in association with a female factor in another 20–30 percent. Although the male factor infertility is traditionally defined by the presence of abnormal semen parameters, it can nowadays be considered even when the seminal analysis is normal but with abnormal functional sperm tests (2).

In the past 20 years, sperm concentration and total sperm count have decreased among young men, male partners in infertile couples, fertile men, and semen donors. In several countries, the sperm concentration levels of several young men have been associated with an increase in time to pregnancy. The reasons for this worsening are poorly established; however, environmental factors are likely to have an impact in this decline (3). The risk factors of male factor infertility may include environmental and lifestyle factors (e.g., smoking, pesticides, radiation, and excessive mobile phone use), local conditions (e.g., varicocele, genitourinary infection, epididymo-orchites, and testicular trauma), and systemic conditions (e.g., diabetes, cancer, medications, and systemic infections). Moreover, the advanced age of the males is associated with a decrease in sperm function and accumulation of sperm genomic damage; male fertility also declines as the male age increases, although not as important as the decline in fecundability with increasing maternal age (1). The same report mentioned that along with this decline observed in the last decades, diagnostic and treatment modalities for infertile men have improved. For instance, physicians now examine not only the traditional semen analysis but also the sperm function and genomic and proteomic expression of seminal plasma proteins; the surgical techniques applied to male infertility problems have also been refined.

In the present chapter, the most recent scientific evidence on male infertility diagnosis and management is reviewed, aiming for the individualized management of infertile patients and an improvement of reproductive outcomes.

5.2 Sperm Physiology and Sperm DNA Integrity

Understanding the sperm physiology and the adequate functioning of the hypothalamic-pituitary-gonadal (HPG) axis is critical for the assessment and management of infertile male patients. Male fertility in humans depends on the continuous daily production of millions of spermatozoa and on adequate spermatogenesis and steroidogenesis. Spermatogenesis is a highly efficient and coordinated process that deals with the production and development of spermatozoa. The entire spermatogenic process requires approximately 74 days, but a more recent study concluded that the total time to produce sperm in normal men might vary between 42 and 76 days, taking approximately 64 days. Every 16 days, a new group of spermatogonia enters the spermatogenic process (4). Spermatogenesis depends on the proper functioning of the HPG axis, which is regulated through the release of gonadotropin-releasing hormone (GnRH). Hypothalamic neurons secrete GnRH in a pulsatile form. Then, GnRH is transported to the anterior compartment of the pituitary gland where it will bind to specific receptors located in the gonadotrophic cells to modulate the synthesis and secretion of pituitary gonadotropins, namely, the follicle-stimulating hormone (FSH) and luteinizing hormones (LH). These hormones are secreted into the systemic circulation and act on the testes. While FSH acts via receptors located in the Sertoli cells, LH stimulates the Leydig cells to produce testosterone, which is an essential prerequisite for male fertility and maintenance of spermatogenesis. Subsequently, steroids and gonadal peptides are secreted and transported to the systemic circulation to modulate the secretion of hypothalamic and pituitary hormones. Thus, spermatogenesis depends on the high levels of intratesticular testosterone and FSH stimulation of the Sertoli cells (5).

Spermatogenesis is classically divided into the following three phases: (1) proliferative or mitotic phase – the primitive germ cells/spermatogonia pass through a series of mitotic divisions, forming new stem cells or cells that will produce the spermatocytes; (2) meiotic phase – the spermatocytes pass through two consecutive divisions producing the spermatids (haploid cells); and (3) spermiogenesis – spermatids differentiate into spermatozoa (6). During the spermatogenesis, significant morphological and functional changes occur in the nucleus. In round spermatids, the nucleus is found in a central position; however, as the spermatid lengthens, it moves to a more eccentric position and undergoes a significant condensation, reaching the size of 10 percent of the initial, favoring hydrodynamics of the sperm. The sperm chromatin has a highly organized and compact structure, consisting of DNA and heterogeneous nucleoproteins. At this point, the chromatin is insoluble and condensed. Such chromatin characteristics are essential to protect genetic integrity during the transport of the paternal genome through the male and female reproductive tracts. Chromatin also ensures that the paternal DNA is delivered in the oocyte enabling the adequate fusion of two gametic genomes and allows that the developing embryo correctly expresses the genetic information (6).

Chromatin compaction and nucleoprotein composition change at the molecular level. In round spermatids, nuclear DNA is arranged around nucleosomes that are composed of histones, as well as in other somatic cells. However, in mature spermatozoa, histone is replaced by protamine, which is a small arginine-rich protein. Protamination is responsible for both higher condensation of the sperm DNA and higher resistance to denaturation, considering that protamines have a higher affinity for DNA than histones. Hypotheses were raised for the function of protamines, stated as follows: condenses the spermatic nucleus, transforming into a more compact and hydrodynamic form; protects the genetic code derived from the spermatozoid; participates in the process of maintenance and repair of sperm DNA integrity; and correlates with the spermatic genetic imprint. For a spermatozoon to be fertile, it must be capable of undergoing decondensation at an appropriate time during fertilization. Thus, the normal sperm chromatin structure and the condensation and decondensation processes are essential for sperm fertilizing ability (7).

Protamination of sperm DNA is essential in the compaction of paternal genome during its transportation to the female genital tract; the DNA integrity is also vital for the accurate transmission of paternal genetic information. Furthermore, the importance of DNA integrity in fertilization, early embryo development, implantation, and pregnancy outcomes has been supported by various in vivo and in vitro studies. Alteration in spermatogenesis, varicocele, inflammatory processes, and other issues related to an increase in oxidative stress may be associated with sperm DNA integrity defects, leading to functional modifications in the sperm that may impact the reproductive outcome in a natural or even assisted conception (7).

Finally, the physiologic levels of reactive oxygen species (ROS) are necessary for adequate sperm capacitation and maturation. However, abnormally elevated amounts of ROS may adversely impair and damage the function of several enzymes and induce lipid peroxidation, causing sperm DNA fragmentation (SDF). Natural antioxidants may act as scavengers of excessive ROS, helping in maintaining a natural redox balance. However, when an imbalance occurs due to excessive ROS production or a reduction in antioxidant activity, an excess of oxidative stress (OS) will occur. Regarding the impact of OS on male fertility, the semen samples of infertile men present higher levels of ROS than those of fertile men (1). Sperm DNA damage is deemed promutagenic, leading to mutations after fertilization as the oocyte attempts to repair the DNA damage before initiating the first cleavage. As speculated, these mutations may be responsible for the induction of infertility, miscarriage, childhood cancer in the offspring, and also a higher risk of imprinting diseases but will be fixed in the germline (4).

5.3 Evaluation

When pregnancy has not occurred after 12 months of unprotected intercourse or after 6 months of failed attempts with a >35-year-old female partner, the male partner must undergo screening evaluation as well. When medical history and/or physical findings are related to specific male infertility, these male partners may be evaluated earlier. The male factor infertility investigation aims to determine the following: (1) potentially reversible conditions; (2) irreversible conditions that are amenable to assisted reproductive techniques (ART) using the sperm of the male partner; (3) irreversible conditions that are not amenable to ART, with sperm donor or adoption as alternatives; (4) life-threatening conditions, such as testicular cancer, that may underlie the infertility and require specific medical treatment; and (5) genetic abnormalities that may impact on child's health if ART is to be employed, allowing to perform a genetic counseling. An appropriate male evaluation may allow the couple to better understand the basis of their infertility. Detection of conditions for which no treatment is available will make couples undergo ineffective therapies. At a minimum, the infertility work-up must include a detailed history, physical examination, and two separate semen analyses to identify the risk factors related to male infertility. Thereafter, specific evaluation must be performed according to the findings of the initial evaluation, allowing the identification of wide-ranging causes of male infertility (2).

5.3.1 Semen Analysis

The semen analysis is the cornerstone on the male factor infertility evaluation, and important treatment decisions are based on the results of the semen analysis. This analysis has been standardized by the World Health Organization (WHO). Its latest references were published in 2010, with a manual for the examination and processing of human semen, establishing the reference limits that should be considered normal when performing a semen analysis (8). If the results of semen analysis are normal, a single test is sufficient. When at least two semen analyses exhibited abnormal results, further andrological evaluation is required (8).

When comparing the last three WHO seminal references that were published in 1992, 1999, and 2010, the latest version established new references that are markedly lower than those previously reported (Table 5.1). The most important change in the references is concerning on the criteria for sperm morphology evaluation. In the last two versions, the Tygerberg (Kruger) criteria were used to evaluate morphology. The morphology judged by Kruger's strict criteria correlated with the fertilization potential of the sperm (9). Kruger et al. observed that when the morphology is <14 percent according to their criteria, the fertilization rate per oocyte is impaired compared with higher percentage levels. When normal morphology is <4 percent, fertilization will be severely impaired. In performing classical *in vitro* fertilization (IVF), when the normal morphology was <4 percent, the fertilization rate was 7.6 percent; when the normal morphology range was 4–14 percent, it was 63.9 percent; and when the morphology was >14 percent, it was within the normal range of the IVF laboratory (9).

Although the semen analysis has been standardized by WHO and the 2010 WHO reference values have been used worldwide as reference, numerous concerns regarding these values have been raised. Despite using controlled studies involving couples with known time to pregnancy (lower than 12 months) to establish new limits, these studies are limited in terms of the population (i.e., 1953 semen samples from only seven countries worldwide) analyzed, the methods used for semen evaluation (studies using different morphology criteria), and having only one sample from each patient was evaluated. According to the fifth edition WHO manual for semen analysis, the fifth centile was the power limit of semen characteristics. Thus, for sperm count, the WHO normal value is $15.0 \times 10^6/\text{mL}$. However, if we evaluated the 50th percentile, a value into which 50 percent of the reference population of "fertile" men falls, and the sperm count would increase to $73.0 \times 10^6/\text{mL}$ (10).

Table 5.1 Semen parameters according to World Health Organization references from 1992, 1999, and 2010

	1992	1999	2010
Volume (mL)	≥2	≥2	≥1.5
Count ($10^6/\text{mL}$)	≥20	≥20	≥15
Total count (10^6)	≥40	≥40	≥39
Motility (%)	≥50	≥50	≥40
Progressive (%)	≥25 (a)	≥25 (a)	≥32
Vitality (%)	≥75	≥75	≥58
Morphology (%)	≥30	14 (Tygerberg)	≥4 (Tygerberg)
Leukocytes ($10^6/\text{mL}$)	<1.0	<1.0	<1.0

Note. Boldface indicates the reference values that have been updated from one to the next version of WHO parameters.

5.3.2 Endocrine Evaluation

Although causes of male infertility remain uncommon, hormonal abnormalities of the hypothalamic-pituitary-testicular axis are well recognized. Some clinicians advocate that all infertile patients should undergo endocrine evaluation; however, endocrine disorders are rare in men with normal sperm parameters (2). Thus, the evaluation is indicated for men presenting the following: (1) sperm concentration <10 million/mL; (2) impaired sexual function; or (3) clinical findings suggestive of any endocrinopathy (4). Initially, hormonal evaluation should be performed with serum FSH and total testosterone measurements. When the total testosterone level is <300 ng/mL, additional evaluation must be performed, including a new testosterone measurement, LH, and prolactin (PRL). A normal FSH level does not exclude impairment in spermatogenesis, but markedly elevated FSH levels are indeed associated with abnormal spermatogenesis (2).

5.3.3 Radiographic Tests

Scrotal ultrasound should not be performed as a routine screening procedure, given that most scrotal pathologies can be identified by a careful examination. However, it is indicated in patients with a history of scrotal surgery, difficulty in genital examination that does not allow the adequate evaluation of related genital diseases, and suspected varicocele recurrence. It also must be performed for men presenting with infertility and testicular cancer risk factors, such as cryptorchidism or a previous testicular neoplasm (2, 11).

Transrectal ultrasound (TRUS) is indicated in patients with low semen volume with/without azoospermia, fructose negative, or an acidic semen. TRUS depicting dilated seminal vesicle (>1.5 cm in diameter), dilated ejaculatory ducts (>2 mm in diameter), and/or midline cystic prostatic structures suggests the diagnosis of complete or partial ejaculatory duct obstruction (11).

Pituitary magnetic resonance imaging (MRI) should be performed in cases of true prolactinemia (PRL > 2× normal reference values). Meanwhile, pelvic/scrotum MRI is indicated in cases of equivocal TRUS, suspicious testicular lesion, and undescended testis. Nowadays, vasography has not been often performed, but it can be performed to rule out obstruction; it is also generally performed during a reconstructive surgery (11).

5.3.4 Genetic Evaluation

Genetic abnormalities may be associated with problems in the production and transport of sperm and may be present in the form of chromosomal, genetic, nucleotide, or epigenetic modifications, representing as one of the most clinically important aspects of male factor infertility (4). Karyotype and Y chromosome analysis is recommended in men with nonobstructive azoospermia (NOA) or severe oligozoospermia (<5 million/mL) (2, 8).

Compared with fertile men, patients with NOA or severe oligozoospermia have a higher risk of exhibiting a genetic abnormality. Although many patients with azoospermia and oligozoospermia present with a genetic predisposition to infertility, the cause in most cases remains unknown. Among the known genetic causes of male infertility are numeric and structural chromosomal abnormalities, Y chromosome microdeletions, X-linked inheritance, and autosomal gene mutations (2, 8). The most common sex chromosome abnormality observed in infertile men is Klinefelter syndrome (47, XXY). Autosomal karyotype abnormalities may also be present, and the most common are Robertsonian translocations, reciprocal translocations, paracentric inversions, and marker chromosomes (8).

Moreover, Y chromosome microdeletions are presented anywhere from 1 in 2000 to 1 in 3000 men. However, this incidence increases to rates of around 7 percent among infertile men with severely impaired spermatogenesis and to 16 percent among patients with azoospermia, though marked differences are reported in different areas worldwide. In general, patients having a Y chromosome microdeletion are asymptomatic, though they may manifest a reduced testicular volume. A specific region on the long arm of the Y chromosome (Yq11) contains 26 genes related to spermatogenesis, the so-called azoos-permia factor (AZF) regions. These genes are organized into three distinct locations as follows: the AZFa, AZFb, and AZFc regions. Deletions in these regions, which may occur independently or in association, may lead to severe oligozoospermia or even azoospermia. The effect on spermatogenesis depends on the affected AZF subregions. The most frequent microdeletion subtype is the AZFc region, which accounts for 80 percent of AZF micro-deletions. Furthermore, AZFb occurs in 15 percent of Y chromosome microdeletions, whereas AZFa is rare and accounts for <3 percent. Sperm-retrieval procedures should be avoided in patients with AZFa, and a controversy exists as to whether it should be performed in patients with AZFb and AZFab; additionally, sperm can be found in around 50–70 percent of patients with AZFc (12).

Most men with congenital bilateral absence of vas deferens (CBAVD) present an abnormality of the cystic fibrosis transmembrane conductance regulator (*CFTR*) gene, which is located on chromosome 7. Almost all men with clinical cystic fibrosis have CBAVD, and 80 percent of them manifest *CFTR* gene mutations. However, failure to identify a *CFTR* abnormality in a male patient with CBAVD does not exclude a mutation entirely, considering that 10–40 percent are undetectable using common clinically available methods. These mutations are also increased in men with congenital bilateral obstruction of the epididymis and those with unilateral vasal agenesis. Importantly, before any treatment using sperm from a patient with CBAVD or congenital unilateral absence of the vas deferens, the female partner of such patient can also be tested to exclude the possibility of being a carrier of the same mutation and to determine the risk of conceiving a child affected by cystic fibrosis (2, 13).

5.3.5 SDF Test

Although the sperm with fragmented DNA can efficiently fertilize an egg with the same efficiency as the sperm without DNA fragmentation, SDF negatively affects embryo quality, impairing the embryo development and compromising the integrity of the embryonic genome. Sperm DNA damage is also associated with spontaneous recurrent miscarriage. Conventional semen analysis is slowly giving space to sperm function tests that measure OS and SDF (4, 14). Thus, although conventional semen analysis continues to be the corner-stone on the assessment of male fertility potential, the sperm DNA damage found in sperm function tests in several cases may indicate subfertility despite the semen analysis results (4). According to a recent published clinical practice guideline, the SDF testing should be performed in the following: (1) male patients with risk factors for OS, including lifestyle conditions (e.g., smoking, obesity, and metabolic syndrome), varicocele, genital infections, advanced age, and toxicant exposure (e.g., environmental, licit or illicit drugs, radiation and chemotherapy); (2) after failed intrauterine insemination (IUI), IVF, or ICSI cycles,

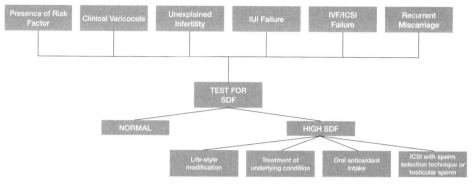

* SDF - Sperm DNA Fragmentation

Figure 5.1 Proposed sperm DNA fragmentation testing and patient management.

provided that no other apparent reasons exist to explain the failure; (3) couples with unexplained infertility; and (4) couples with recurrent miscarriage (Figure 5.1) (7).

Several tests for SDF evaluation have been developed, and the most commonly used tests are the terminal deoxynucleotidyl transferase-mediated dUTP nick end labeling, single-cell gel electrophoresis assay, sperm chromatin dispersion test, and sperm chromatin structure assay. Although the American Society for Reproductive Medicine does not recommend the routinely performance of any of these tests, they agree that the effect of abnormal SDF on the value of IUI or IVF and intracytoplasmic sperm injection (ICSI) results may be clinically informative (2).

5.4 Etiology

The majority of male infertility is idiopathic; for this reason, many patients' abnormalities in sperm parameters or even azoospermia remain unexplained. The known causes of male infertility may be classified as pretesticular, testicular, and posttesticular. *Pretesticular causes* are as follows: (1) hypothalamic disease, including gonadotropin deficiency (Kallmann syndrome), isolated LH deficiency, isolated FSH deficiency, and congenital hypogonadotropic syndromes; and (2) pituitary disease, including pituitary insufficiency, hyperprolactinemia, exogenous hormones, and growth hormone deficiency. *Testicular causes* include the following: (1) nonchromosomal diseases, including varicocele, cryptorchidism, Sertoli cell-only syndrome, chemotherapy, and radiotherapy; and (2) chromosomal diseases, including Klinefelter syndrome, XX male, XYY male, among others. Lastly, *posttesticular causes* are as follows: congenital blockage of the ductal system, cystic fibrosis, acquired blockage of the ductal system, antisperm antibodies, ejaculatory duct obstruction, male accessory gland infection (1).

5.5 Management

In managing male infertility, the underlying specific medical or surgical diagnosis must be focused on. An empiric pharmacologic therapy aiming to improve the spermatogenesis may be implemented, as well as ART to overcome male infertility. All the options and outcomes of each strategy should be presented and discussed with the couples that will select the most affordable treatment to perform. The medical treatment for known causes of male infertility tends to have high success rates. However, empirical treatment is implemented in cases of idiopathic or genetic causes of male infertility, but the results are controversial (5).

5.5.1 Empirical Treatment

The use of gonadotropins in men with idiopathic infertility is rarely reported. However, some recent studies have shown that their use can optimize the chances of sperm retrieval in patients submitted to testicular sperm extraction procedures. Currently, the use of gonadotropins empirically in cases of oligospermia and azoospermia lacks consensus (5).

Currently, the use of antioxidants in the treatment of male infertility is not specifically recommended. Their use is completely empirical (5). In the most recent review on the use of antioxidants for treating male subfertility, antioxidants may improve live birth rates for couples attending fertility clinics. However, these data are from small randomized studies, making the quality of evidence equivocal. The current evidence is inconclusive according to the serious risk of bias in the studies evaluating their use. Thus, although the use of antioxidants might improve sperm quality by reducing the oxidative damage for sperm, further well-designed studies reporting on pregnancy and live births are required to elucidate the exact role of antioxidants in treating male infertility (15).

5.5.2 Hormonal Therapy

Although testosterone is fundamentally important for spermatogenesis, the administration of testosterone or other androgens should be avoided. They act in a negative feedback on HPG and present a contraceptive effect because they inhibit the LH stimulation of intra-testicular testosterone production and also the FSH stimulation of the Sertoli cells (5).

The pulsatile administration of GnRH is an effective treatment to replace GnRH deficiency due to hypogonadotropic hypogonadism (HH) in infertile men. It is effective in inducing spermatogenesis as early as 4 months after therapy initiation, inducing spermatogenesis in approximately 85 percent of patients. On average, 60 percent of couples will achieve pregnancy after 9 months of treatment, if no association of female factors of infertility exists. However, pulsatile GnRH treatment is limited by availability, inconvenience of delivery by carrying a pump, and the need to regularly change subcutaneous needles (5).

In men with pituitary insufficiency, the testosterone production cannot be induced by pulsatile GnRH, and the treatment is based on gonadotropins to stimulate the spermatogenesis and testosterone production. The gonadotropins can also be used in men with HH. Initially, hCG is solely administered at 1500–2500 IU twice weekly. After several months of treatment, if adequate levels of testosterone are achieved but no sperm is found in semen analysis, FSH can be introduced. The doses may range from 75–150 IU of FSH or human menopausal gonadotropin (hMG) two to three times weekly. Gonadotropins induce spermatogenesis in 80 percent of men; however, the treatment duration may vary from 6 months to 24 months. In general, the therapy is well tolerated, and the dose can be adjusted to adequately control the testosterone levels, thereby minimizing the side effects (5).

Aromatase inhibitors (AI) have been used as an off-label treatment in men with oligoastenozoospermia (OAT) and azoospermia. The rationale of its administration is to increase the testosterone levels and decrease the estrogen levels, and to inhibit the peripheral metabolism of testosterone. Reducing the estrogenic effect (given that high levels of estrogen are associated with low testosterone levels) impairs spermatogenesis adequately. For estrogen reduction, 1 mg of anastrozole daily or 2.5 mg of letrozole daily can be used. Nowadays, either of these drugs is used in OAT or azoospermia presenting with testosterone levels < 300 ng/dL with Testosterone/Estradiol (T/E) ratio < 10:1 (5).

Selective estrogen receptor modulators (SERMs), such as clomiphene citrate (CC) and tamoxifen, are other off-label drugs that have been used to treat male infertility. As the SERMs inhibit central estrogen feedback and upregulates LH and FSH production, testicular testosterone is effectively produced, leading to the induction of spermatogenesis. However, the benefit of empirical therapy for idiopathic male infertility remains controversial (5).

5.5.3   Varicocele

Varicocele is the dilatation of the pampiniform plexus veins. It is a common condition both in men with normal spermatogenesis and in men with abnormal semen parameters. It is the most common cause of male infertility, affecting approximately 15–20 percent of the general population. Around 35–40 percent of men have primary infertility, and up to 80 percent of men have secondary infertility. Despite being more common on the left side, varicoceles are found bilaterally in up to 50 percent of the patients. It rarely occurs on the right side alone; when it occurs, further investigation is necessary for the presence of situs inversus, retroperitoneal tumors, and insertion of the spermatic vein into the right renal vein. The prevalence of varicocele is low among boys aged 2–10 years, and it becomes relatively high in adolescents and adults, suggesting that venous incompetence primarily occurs during testicular growth. Although its physiopathology has been discussed for over 50 years, the exact mechanism that would lead to infertility has remained unknown. However, the most commonly accepted mechanisms include hyperthermia and testicular tissue hypoxia or ischemia, leading to alteration in conventional semen parameters and of sperm function tests, such as OS and SDF (11, 16, 17). Varicocele may also be associated with failure of ipsilateral testicular growth and development, pain and discomfort symptoms and hypogonadism (8).

Varicocele diagnosis is based primarily on physical examination; imaging studies are only indicated when physical examination is inconclusive or in cases of recurrence after a previous repair. Only clinically palpable varicocele has been clearly associated with infertility (18). The most widely used classification is the Dubin grading system, which classifies varicocele on a scale of 1 to 3, with grade 3 being present on visual inspection of the scrotum, grade 2 being easily palpable, and grade 1 only being palpable with Valsalva maneuver (19).

Varicocele can impair spermatogenesis through several distinct pathophysiological mechanisms, such as scrotal hyperthermia, hormonal disturbances, testicular hypoperfusion, hypoxia, and toxic metabolite backflow. Current evidence supports OS as a key element in the pathophysiology of varicocele-related infertility. Both ROS and apoptosis markers increase in the semen of infertile men with varicocele (20). Despite the ROS plays an important physiological role in fertility, they are involved in the process of sperm capacitation, acrosome reaction, hyperactivation, and sperm–oocyte fusion. When an imbalance between ROS production and antioxidant protection occurs or when the antioxidant capacity is reduced, OS may be present, leading to damage in normal spermatozoa. Thus, one of the key elements of varicocele-induced infertility is OS, which appears when the production of potentially destructive ROS exceeds the natural antioxidant defenses, leading to cellular damage (20). The ROS is released in men with varicocele under heat and hypoxic stress through the following three components: the principal cells in the epididymis, the endothelial cells in the dilated pampiniform plexus, and the testicular cells. Consequently, the sperm membrane is damaged, affecting both sperm motility and sperm–oocyte fusion. Furthermore, OS may negatively affect the sperm chromatin by inducing breaks in the DNA strands (11). Notwithstanding, the reasons why some patients with varicocele are infertile while most are not, remain unclear. Probably, the presence of intrinsic mechanisms to counteract the action of ROS may explain why most patients with varicocele retain their fertility (17).

In treating varicocele, the following should be considered: (1) presence of a palpable (clinical) varicocele; (2) the couple has known infertility; (3) the female partner has normal fertility or a potentially treatable cause of infertility; and (4) the male partner has abnormal semen parameters. The current options for varicocele management may involve its repair, intrauterine insemination, and IVF/ICSI. In order to reach a consensus, many factors may be taken in account, and all the factors must be discussed with the couple. The improvement in semen parameters after varicocele repair may take 3–6 months. The varicocele repair is not indicated in patients with a subclinical varicocele (i.e., those only identified when performing an ultrasound and not clinical examination). It is associated with a low risk of complications; in most studies, semen parameters and fertility improved after repair. IVF may be considered instead of treating the varicocele when ART is necessary to treat a female factor, regardless of the presence of varicocele and abnormal semen parameters (18). Thus, adequate evaluation of the couple is fundamental to establish the most suitable treatment for them.

The surgical repair is the most accepted approach for varicocele treatment. Percutaneous embolization is also an alternative, mainly in cases of recurrence after the surgical approach. Different surgical approaches include conventional retroperitoneal, laparoscopic/robotic, inguinal, or microsurgical inguinal or subinguinal. The "gold standard" approach is the microsurgical subinguinal, which is associated with a lower risk of recurrence and hydrocele formation. Varicocele repair is associated with improvements in conventional semen parameters and on SDF, and it has been recently indicated for patients with hypogonadism. Moreover, the benefit in performing the repair in NOA cases has been recently debated, given that NOA can return the sperm in the ejaculate or at least lead to an increase in sperm-retrieval rates when performing testicular biopsy in these cases (11).

5.5.4 Azoospermia

Azoospermia is defined by the absence of sperm in the ejaculate, occurring in 1 percent of the male population and up to 15 percent of infertile patients. This condition is based on the examination of multiple semen specimens, considering that transitory azoospermia may occur due to toxic, environmental, infectious, or iatrogenic conditions (21). Furthermore, it can be classified into the following three categories: 1. pretesticular, including endocrine abnormalities having adverse effects on spermatogenesis (secondary testicular failure); 2. testicular (primary testicular failures), encompassing spermatogenic disorders intrinsic to the testes; 3. posttesticular, related to ejaculatory dysfunction or ductal obstruction that impairs the adequate transit of sperm (13).

In the clinical practice, the azoospermia is distinguished into two categories, namely, obstructive azoospermia (OA) and NOA. Up to 2/3 of patients with azoospermia have been associated with a spectrum of untreatable testicular disorders leading to spermatogenic failure (21). In differentiating OA from NOA, important information such as history, physical examination, and laboratory assessment results can be utilized. Together, these parameters provide >90 percent prediction of whether the condition is an OA or a NOA. In general, a patient with NOA has normal semen volume (>1.5 mL) and pH (>7.2), indicating that both seminal vesicles and patent ejaculatory ducts are functional. Proper laboratory techniques for semen analysis are crucial to reduce errors and improve the precision when interpreting the results (21). Although rarely performed as a diagnostic purpose, testicular biopsy can accurately differentiate OA from NOA (11). The differentiation between OA and NOA is crucial, given that OA presents a favorable prognosis because spermatogenesis is not disrupted compared with NOA; NOA is associated with a spectrum of various serious and untreatable conditions related to intrinsic testicular impairment (21).

5.5.4.1 NOA

Men with suspected NOA should undergo adequate hormonal and genetic evaluation that will provide important information for preparing for sperm-retrieval procedures or even for hormonal therapy, such as in HH (11). The HH is a rare endocrine disorder in which a lack of appropriate stimulation by gonadotropins results in spermatogenic failure. It is easily recognized, given that patients with HH have remarkably low levels of pituitary gonadotropins and androgens (FSH and LH < 1.2 IU/mL, testosterone levels < 300 ng/dL) (21). Patients with HH may avoid sperm-retrieval procedures when using gonadotropins (presented in Section 5.5.2), considering that they generally respond to hormone replacement, although it may take up to 6 months of treatment to identify sperm in the ejaculate (11).

The management of patients with NOA may be based on the following steps: 1. differential diagnosis of azoospermia and conformation that NOA is due to spermatogenic failure; 2. counseling about the chances of finding sperm for ICSI; 3. evaluating potential candidates for using adjunct therapies before performing sperm-retrieval procedures; 4. use of the most effective and efficient strategy for recovering sperm in a testicular procedure; 5. use of the most appropriate technique for handling the testicular tissue, increasing the chance of finding sperm for ICSI (21).

In patients with NOA, genetic abnormalities are prevalent, and the most common sex chromosome abnormality detected in men with NOA is the Klinefelter syndrome. AZF microdeletions should also be tested because it will not only offer a cause for the azoospermia but also relate to the prognosis of the surgical sperm retrieval. Sperm retrieval should not be offered to patients with AZFa, AZFb, or AZFa/b microdeletions due to an extremely low chance of retrieving sperm (11). Other common etiology conditions related to NOA are congenital abnormalities (cryptorchidism), postinfection (orchitis), gonadotoxin exposure (radiotherapy/chemotherapy), testicular trauma, and idiopathy (21).

Nowadays, the insight into whether the use of hormonal therapies previously from the sperm-retrieval procedure may have an impact on the retrieval rates is highly controversial. Pretreatment with CC, AI, and gonadotropins seems to improve the sperm-retrieval rates (11). Their use may be beneficial in increasing intratesticular testosterone levels and normalizing estrogen levels prior to semen retrieval. However, the population that may benefit from their use aiming to optimize the sperm-retrieval rates is yet to be established, given that no randomized studies have evaluated the use of medical therapies prior to sperm-retrieval (5).

At present, men with NOA associated with unilateral or bilateral varicoceles represent a management dilemma. Although many other factors (e.g., genetic etiologies) may be related to azoospermia, the varicocele may be the only factor related to NOA. As shown in selected patients, varicocele repair may be associated with sperm returning to the ejaculate to various degrees in 10–40 percent of patients. In those patients that continue without sperm in the ejaculate, the varicocele repair may be related to an increase in the likelihood of sperm retrieval when performing a testicular biopsy (13).

The surgical sperm-retrieval procedures and the ICSI have significantly changed the perspectives of men who were previously diagnosed as sterile. Multiple refinements have been introduced into the sperm-retrieval procedures, in the surgical procedure, and in the laboratory handling the extracted material, but the most important was the introduction of surgical microscopy (11). Sperm-retrieval procedures aim to offer the highest chance of obtaining an adequate number of sperm to be used in an ICSI procedure or to be cryopreserved, with the minimal risk of testicular damage to maintain androgen activity and the chances of success if repeated procedures are necessary in the future (21). In NOA cases, the sperm can be retrieved percutaneously (testicular sperm aspiration), with a conventional open testicular biopsy (testicular sperm extraction, TESE) or with the use of a microscope (micro TESE) aiming to identify larger seminiferous tubules that would be associated with a higher chance of having sperm inside (11). Overall, sperm is found in around 50–60 percent of patients with NOA. These rates are related to the sperm-retrieval procedure implemented and to the testicular histology related to azoospermia. Sperm can be found in up to 90 percent of patients with hypospermatogenesis, up to 50 percent of those with maturation arrest, and around 10–20 percent of those with Sertoli cell-only syndrome.

5.5.4.2 OA

OA occurs in up to 40 percent of men with azoospermia and is related to the absence of spermatozoa and spermatogenic cells in semen and postejaculate urine due to obstruction. Obstruction may be congenital or acquired. Congenital causes of OA include CBAVD, unilateral vasal agenesis, ejaculatory duct obstruction, and idiopathic epididymal obstruction. Acquired causes of OA include vasectomy, infection, trauma, or an iatrogenic injury (22). In general, men with OA exhibit normal testes size, epididymal enlargement, and normal FSH levels. In addition, it can be related to intratesticular, epididymal, vas deferens, and ejaculatory duct obstructions (8). Patients with ejaculatory duct obstruction generally have a low semen volume, acidic pH, and absence of fructose. These patients should undergo differential diagnosis to exclude the possibility of retrograde ejaculation, with the performance of a postejaculate urine analysis. When they do not have a retrograde ejaculation and the semen pH is less than 7.2, a TRUS can be performed to evaluate the dilation of seminal vesicles or ejaculatory ducts. Low ejaculate volume not related to hypogonadism or CBAVD is most likely caused by ejaculatory duct obstruction, although it can also be related to ejaculatory dysfunction (13).

The CBAVD and unilateral vasal agenesis is demonstrated by physical examination, and the normal vasa can be easily palpated within the scrotum. Around 25 percent of men with unilateral vasal agenesis and 10–15 percent of patients with CBAVD have unilateral renal agenesis that can be detected by ultrasound. In patients with unilateral vasal agenesis, renal agenesis is not associated with CFTR mutation and may be explained by different genetic mutations that lead to anomalies in the Wolffian duct with subsequent abnormalities in the seminal vesicles, vas deferens, and epididymis (13).

In patients with OA, both reconstructive surgery and sperm-retrieval procedures combined with IVF/ICSI can be performed. In cases of planning a reconstructive surgery, performing an adequate evaluation of the female partner is fundamentally important to exclude any cause of female infertility. The costs and success rates of each strategy must be present and discussed with the couple. Several factors may be related to the choice of treatment, but ultimately the choice must be based on the couple's preference (22).

In cases of vasectomy, up to 8 percent of patients will have the desire to father a child after performing vasectomy. In cases in which association of a female factor is not found and the solely responsible for the infertility is the OA, vasectomy reversal may be an option. In experienced hands, the reversal success rates with return of sperm to the ejaculate may be found in 45–98 percent of patients, depending on the time (years) between the vasectomy and the reversal procedure. Moreover, up to 65–75 percent of couples may achieve pregnancy without ART (22). Thus, the vasectomy reversal must be discussed with the couples, mainly those without advanced reproductive female age in which ART procedure delay will not affect the chances of delivery in the near future.

In general, the sperm-retrieval procedures in OA are minimally invasive and present a low complication risk; successful sperm retrieval should be expected in most patients (22). The retrieval procedures can be performed percutaneously from epididymis (percutaneous epididymal sperm aspiration) or with the use of a surgery microscope (microsurgical epididymal sperm aspiration). If the epididymal procedure fails in retrieving sperm, testicular sperm retrieval can be performed (11). If the female partner can naturally conceive, patients with ejaculatory duct obstruction may perform a transurethral resection of ejaculatory ducts, which can improve sperm quality in 70–80 percent (11).

5.5.5 High SDF

Patients with high SDF levels have several available treatment options, including risk factor modification, frequent ejaculation, antioxidant therapy, varicocele correction, use of sperm selection techniques for ICSI, and use of testicular sperm for ICSI (11).

Lifestyle factors, such as smoking and exposure to environmental/occupational chemicals, obesity, and advanced paternal age, have a negative impact on sperm DNA quality and are related to SDF. Thus, patients need to be counseled on changes in lifestyle. However, further research is required to determine if these changes may translate into better reproductive outcomes (23).

The current evidence supports OS as a central element in the pathophysiology of varicocele-induced infertility. Varicocele repair may alleviate OS and reduce SDF, leading to improved fertility both natural and assisted. Thus, infertility practitioners should advise men with clinical varicocele on the correlation between sperm DNA damage and OS and discuss varicocele repair as a way for reducing SDF and potentially improving fertility (24, 25).

Although SDF is related to an imbalance in oxidative and antioxidative parameters, the benefits of antioxidants are not universal. When the antioxidant therapy is planned, it is given for approximately 3 months, and its effect on SDF is evaluated with SDF testing. The ideal candidates for antioxidant therapy and the optimal regimen, dosage, and duration are still unknown (23).

When performing ART, sperm selection techniques may be employed, aiming to overcome SDF. Various techniques to select sperm with lower DNA damage have been proposed, although no single strategy is clearly related to improvements in ART outcomes. Recently, the use of testicular sperm in preference over ejaculated sperm has gained increased attention, owing to reports of better ICSI outcomes, which are mainly related to a decrease in miscarriage rates. The biological plausibility for using testicular sperm is that decreased DNA fragmentation levels are observed in testicular sperm compared with using ejaculated sperm. The oxidative induced damage to sperm DNA integrity, related to the sperm transport through the seminiferous tubules and epididymis, could be bypassed using the testicular sperm. Thus, this approach is an option to be discussed with patients in which SDF levels remain high despite treating the underlying conditions or without an apparent factor related to the high SDF. However, the benefits and risks of this strategy have to be balanced, given that clinical evidence supporting the use of testicular sperm instead of ejaculated sperm in ICSI cycles is still limited (23).

5.6 Conclusion

Considering that the male factor infertility is present in 40–50 percent of the infertile couples, its management should be performed in coordination with the female manage-ment. Hence, an adequate counseling of the couple regarding the treatment options and chances should take place. However, high-quality studies that evaluate and compare different treatment strategies involving male factor infertility are still unavailable, and many treatments are implemented empirically. Nevertheless, an increasing body of evidence exists wherein the ART based on the female infertility etiology is the only option for the couple, and an adequate evaluation of the male factor may be related to improved ART outcomes. The infertile couple should be considered and treated in unity, aiming in offering the most effective, safe, and suitable treatment for each couple and also for the offspring.

References

1. Agarwal A, Majzoub A, Parekh N, et al. A schematic overview of the current status of male infertility practice. World J Mens Health 2019;37. doi:10.5534/wjmh.190068.

2. Diagnostic evaluation of the infertile male: a committee opinion. Fertil Steril 2015;103 (3):e18–25.

3. Virtanen HE, Jørgensen N, Toppari J. Semen quality in the 21st century. Nat Rev Urol 2017;14(2): 120–130.

4. Esteves SC, Agarwal A. Novel concepts in male infertility. Int Braz J Urol 2011;37 (1):5–15.

5. Dabaja AA, Schlegel PN. Medical treatment of male infertility. Transl Androl Urol 2014;3(1):8.

6. Neto FTL, Bach PV, Najari BB, et al. Spermatogenesis in humans and its affecting factors. Semin Cell Dev Biol 2016;59:10–26.

7. Agarwal A, Cho C-L, Majzoub A, et al. The Society for Translational Medicine: clinical practice guidelines for sperm DNA fragmentation testing in male infertility. Transl Androl Urol 2017;6(S4):S720–733.

8. Jungwirth A, Giwercman A, Tournaye H, et al. European Association of Urology Guidelines on Male Infertility: the 2012 update. Eur Urol 2012;62(2):324–332.

9. Kruger TF, Acosta AA, Simmons KF, et al. Predictive value of abnormal sperm morphology in in vitro fertilization. Fertil Steril 1988;49(1):112–117.

10. Esteves SC, Zini A, Aziz N, et al. Critical appraisal of World Health Organization's new reference values for human semen characteristics and effect on diagnosis and treatment of subfertile men. Urology 2012;79 (1):16–22.

11. Agarwal A, Majzoub A, Parekh N, et al. A schematic overview of the current status of male infertility practice. World J Mens Health 2019;37. doi:10.5534/ wjmh.190068.

12. Management of nonobstructive azoospermia: a committee opinion. Fertil Steril 2018;110(7):1239–1245.

13. Hwang K, Smith JF, Coward RM, et al. Evaluation of the azoospermic male: a committee opinion. Fertil Steril 2018;109 (5):777–782.

14. Esteves SC. Novel concepts in male factor infertility: clinical and laboratory perspectives. J Assist Reprod Genet 2016;33 (10):1319–1335.

15. Smits RM, Mackenzie-Proctor R, Yazdani A, et al. Antioxidants for male subfertility. Cochrane Database Syst Rev 2019;3:CD007411. doi:10.1002/14651858. CD007411.pub4.

16. Jensen CFS, Østergren P, Dupree JM, et al. Varicocele and male infertility. Nat Rev Urol 2017;14(9):523–533.

17. Esteves SC, Agarwal A. Afterword to varicocele and male infertility: current concepts and future perspectives. Asian J Androl 2016;18(2):319–322. doi:10.4103/ 1008-682X.172820.

18. Report on varicocele and infertility: a committee opinion. Fertil Steril 2014;102 (6):1556–1560.

19. Miyaoka R, Esteves SC. A critical appraisal on the role of varicocele in male infertility. Adv Urol 2012;2012:1–9.

20. Agarwal A, Hamada A, Esteves SC. Insight into oxidative stress in varicocele-associated male infertility: part 1. Nat Rev Urol 2012;9(12):678–690.

21. Esteves S. Clinical management of infertile men with nonobstructive azoospermia. Asian J Androl 2015;17(3):459–470.

22. The management of obstructive azoospermia: a committee opinion. Fertil Steril 2019;111(5):873–880.

23. Esteves SC. Interventions to prevent sperm DNA damage effects on reproduction. Adv Exp Med Biol 2019;1166:119–148. doi:10.1007/978-3-030-21664-1_8.

24. Esteves SC, Santi D, Simoni M. An update on clinical and surgical interventions to reduce sperm DNA fragmentation in infertile men. Andrology 2019;6: andr.12724.

25. Roque M, Esteves SC. Effect of varicocele repair on sperm DNA fragmentation: a review. Int Urol Nephrol 2018;50 (4):583–603.

6 Individualized Fertilization Technique in the IVF Laboratory
IVF or ICSI?

Neelke De Munck and Ibrahim Elkhatib

6.1 History of IVF and ICSI

The history of in vitro fertilization (IVF) and embryo transfer (ET) goes back to the early 1890s when Walter Heape, a professor and physician at the University of Cambridge, England, reported the first known case of embryo transplantation in rabbits, long before the applications to human fertility were even suggested. In 1934 Pincus and Enzmann, from the Laboratory of General Physiology at Harvard University, published a paper in the Proceedings of the National Academy of Sciences of the USA, raising the possibility that mammalian oocytes can undergo normal development in vitro. Two decades later, in 1948, Miriam Menken and John Rock retrieved more than 800 oocytes from women during operations for various conditions. One hundred thirty-eight of these oocytes were exposed to spermatozoa in vitro, and they published their experiences in the American Journal of Obstetrics and Gynecology.

The first mammalian (rabbit) life birth after IVF was reported by Chang and colleagues in 1959. Fertilization was induced by the incubation of ovulated oocytes with capacitated sperm in a small Carrel flask for four hours. This achievement paved the way for human reproductive technologies. It took more than two decades before the first human IVF pregnancy was reported by the Monash research team of Professors Carl Wood and John Leeton in Melbourne, Australia. Unfortunately, this resulted in an early miscarriage.

Professionals in the fields of microscopy, embryology, and anatomy laid the foundations for future achievements. Through the years, numerous modifications have been made in the development of human IVF: refinement of fertilization and embryo culture media, improvements in equipment and cleanroom conditions, embryo biopsy, and genetic testing. The world's first B2 culture medium, known as "the French medium," was developed by Menezo in 1976. This specific medium reflected the follicular, tubal, and uterine environments of the sheep, rabbits, and humans.

Prior to 1978, women with defected fallopian tubes were considered to be sterile by their physicians. At least one functional fallopian tube is necessary for natural fertilization of an oocyte by sperm in vivo. Physicians often performed reparative surgeries for the defective tubes as an endeavor of restoring fertility. IVF was considered experimental, was not applied clinically and resulted in miscarriages whenever attempted. Not until the late 1970s when a patient of nine years of primary infertility due to tubal occlusion named Lesley Brown, was treated by Patrick Steptoe and Robert Edwards. She underwent laparoscopic single oocyte retrieval, that was fertilized in the laboratory and later transferred on day 2.5 as an eight-cell embryo into the uterus and resulted in the first live birth from IVF on July 25, 1978, Louise Brown (1).

In the mid-1980s new techniques were developed to increase the success rate after embryo transfer. One of these techniques was referred to as gamete intrafallopian transfer (GIFT) in which oocytes are retrieved laparoscopically, followed by immediate replacement of the oocytes and sperm in the fallopian tubes. Despite the fact that GIFT increased the success rates, patients with severe male factor, tubal occlusion, or pelvic adhesions could not benefit from this technique. Another technique arose in that period called zygote intrafallopian transfer (ZIFT) where oocytes were retrieved laparoscopically, fertilized in vitro and transferred into the fallopian tubes at the pronuclear stage. While ZIFT allowed the confirmation of fertilization, the use of two laparoscopies, one for oocyte retrieval and the other for zygote transfer, was a major limitation of this approach (2).

In 1987 transvaginal follicle aspiration was introduced, this method of follicle aspiration became the procedure of choice due to better visualization, precise control, and less patient discomfort (3). Infertility treatment regimens became more dependent on conventional IVF, however, there was still a limitation in the treatment of male factor infertility, whether it was due to a lower sperm count (oligozoospermia), sperm motility (asthenozoospermia), morphology (teratozoospermia), or even azoospermic males. Several procedures were developed in the eighties in order to improve the success rate and to compensate the compromised outcome in cases of male factor infertility. The first procedure was partial zona dissection (PZD) where a small opening was made in the zona pellucida to enhance sperm penetration (4). Another technique was subzonal insemination (SUZI) where few motile sperm were microinjected in the perivitelline space. The results of these techniques were not satisfactory, were inconsistent, and were of limited use in cases of severe male infertility. The work of Gianpiero Palermo was dedicated to improving fertilization especially in cases of severe male infertility. Palermo exposed sperm cells to follicular fluid to enhance acrosome reaction (5) and reported a fertilization rate of 40 percent using SUZI when adequate number of sperm cells were available but failed to achieve the same outcome in cases of severe male factor cases. To overcome the low fertilization in severe male factor cases, Palermo decided to further enhance the interaction between the sperm cell and the oocyte by releasing the sperm in a cleft in the oolema. While performing this procedure, in some cases unintentionally the membrane was pierced, and the spermatozoon was released in the ooplasm. He noticed that almost whenever this incident happens the oocyte got fertilized. Palermo shared his observation with Hubert Joris, a technician who was working with him, who recalled a case where the only fertilized oocyte was the one pierced accidently through the membrane, and the resulting embryo was transferred and achieved a pregnancy.

The technique of intracytoplasmic sperm injection (ICSI) where a single sperm is injected directly into the oocyte's cytoplasm was one of the biggest achievements in the field of reproductive medicine, introduced in 1992 by Palermo and Van Steirteghem (6). Fertilization rates of 60–70 percent were reported using ICSI, which was a significant improvement compared to other techniques such as SUZI and PZD. From that day onward, ICSI could successfully be applied in cases of severe male factor and surgically retrieved sperm.

6.2 Natural Conception

Fertilization is a complex process that leads to the union of the male and female germ cells to produce a zygote. Fertilization only occurs after both the sperm cell and the oocyte complete their cytoplasmic and nuclear maturation. In nature, normal fertilization involves several essential consecutive steps:

- ovulation
- introduction of adequate number of motile sperm within the vagina
- sperm capacitation
- sperm interaction with the cumulus cells
- sperm penetration of the zona pellucida
- sperm–oocyte fusion
- oocyte activation
- pronucleus formation
- syngamy

Pituitary gonadotropins act on large antral follicles and initiate the resumption of meiosis for oocytes arrested at prophase of meiosis I. The cumulus oophorus starts to expand in preparation for ovulation, these sticky cells will aid in the oocyte-sperm interaction as well as the uptake by the human oviduct fimbriae. Semen is disposed near the cervical os and sperm will start swimming into the cervical canal, which will coagulate within minutes of coitus by forming a loose gel structure made of structural proteins (Semenogelin I and II). Prostate-specific antigen, which is an enzyme secreted by the prostate gland, will degrade the gel coagulum after 30–60 minutes. The coagulum protects the sperm from vaginal acidic environment and immunological responses that can damage the sperm. The sperm traverse the cervical canal and will exit the uterine cavity into the isthmus of the oviduct. Out of the millions of sperm disposed in the anterior vagina, only a few thousand reach the oviducts, and only hundreds make it to the site of fertilization, the ampulla region, which can be thought of as a natural selection of the fittest and most suitable sperm to achieve fertilization.

Sperm capacitation is a combination of processes that alter the sperm cell structure to enable them to undergo the acrosome reaction and result in obtaining fertilization competence. These processes involve alteration of the membrane proteins and lipids to get rid of the inhibitory factors, changes in the intracellular pH, calcium concentration, and cAMP-dependent protein tyrosine phosphorylation and dephosphorylation. Human sperm capacitation starts as soon as the sperm is ejaculated and takes around six hours. In vitro, capacitation can be induced by the removal of the seminal plasma during a swim-up procedure or gradient and incubating the spermatozoa in a bicarbonate-buffered solution containing electrolytes, metabolic energy sources, and protein source, at 37°–39°C. The acrosome represents the anterior region of the sperm head, and contains several enzymes including hyaluronidase, acrosin, collagenase, phospholipase C, and arylsulfatase. The spermatozoa traverse the cumulus oophorus by utilizing its motility and with the help of enzyme hyaluronidase that is either present on the sperm plasma membrane or from the sperm acrosome. The sperm then reaches the zona pellucida (ZP) which triggers the acrosome reaction process, causing changes in the sperm plasma membrane permeability and intracellular ions concentration. The oocyte ZP is an acellular glycoprotein that is composed of four glycoproteins: ZP1, ZP2, ZP3, and ZP4 that are encoded by genes on chromosomes 11, 16, 7, and 1, respectively. The capacitated sperm bind to both ZP3 and ZP4 inducing the acrosome reaction marked by the fusion of the outer acrosomal membrane and the sperm head plasma membrane allowing its content to be released. The acrosome-reacted sperm then binds to ZP2 and releases enzymes such as acrosin and lysins that dissolve the ZP.

Once the sperm is through the ZP, it binds to the oolemma and induces the cortical reaction. Cortical granules are membrane-bound organelles containing enzymes and muco-polysaccharides. When the sperm penetrates the ZP, the cortical granules fuse with the oocyte plasma membrane and release their content into the perivitelline space by exocytosis, causing hardening of the ZP, and the oocyte plasma membrane becomes a mosaic of cortical granule membrane and original plasma membrane. The cortical reaction process also induces the hydrolysis of ZP sperm receptors which is essential in the block to polyspermy.

Oocyte activation is marked by the cortical granule exocytosis and resumption of meiosis. After the sperm penetrates the oolemma the sperm postacrosomal region fuses with the oocytes' microvillus surface. The sperm introduces soluble cytosolic factor, phospholipase C zeta, into the oocyte cytoplasm which triggers the oocyte activation via inositol 1,4,5-tripho-sphate pathway (IP_3), which triggers the calcium oscillations. The sperm nucleus contains chromatin that is tightly packed with highly charged amino acids called protamines, which are responsible for condensing the DNA and repressing transcription. Extensive disulfide bonds between protamines make the sperm head rigid which is important for zona pellucida penetration. When the sperm nucleus enters the oocyte cytoplasm, the disulfide bonds between the protamines are reduced by oocyte-derived glutathione. Another molecule is required to replace the protamines with oocyte histones, data suggest that this molecule is heparin sulfate. The sperm nuclear envelope breaks down and the highly condensed chromatin disperse so that chromatin filaments are released into the cytoplasm.

The sperm enters the oocyte when it is in metaphase II stage, during the sperm chromatin decondensation, as described above, the oocyte enters the telophase II. During telophase II sperm chromatin decondensation is completed, protamines replaced by his-tones and the male and female pronuclear envelops develop synchronously. During oogen-esis the oocyte loses both centrioles and does not exhibit granular perinuclear centrosomal material, while during spermatogenesis there is partial loss of male centrosomes when the spermatids transform into mature sperm. The proximal centriole remains intact, though inactive, while the distal centriole aids in the formation of sperm axoneme and doesn't function as centriole. After fertilization an active zygotic centrosome is formed, with some maternal input around the sperm centriole, which duplicates at the pronuclear stage and forms sperm aster. The formed sperm aster is essential for pronuclear development, migration of pronuclei toward syngamy and the formation of the mitotic spindles.

The two pronuclei (PN) formed in the zygote contain nuclear precursor bodies (NPBs), their number and arrangement can be used as an indicator of embryonic development potential (7). The NPBs migrate and merge to form the nucleoli in a time dependent manner. The pre-RNA synthesis in the nucleoli is important for translational processes when the embryonic genome is activated.

The last step of fertilization process before the first cleavage is called syngamy. After the formation of the male and female pronucleus, they start to gradually migrate toward the center of the oocyte. The chromatin of each PN rotates to face each other placing the centrosome between them. The nuclear envelops dissolve few hours before the first mitotic division and the two sets of chromosomes from each PN pair in syngamy, align on the newly formed mitotic spindles and are ready for segregation during the first mitotic division.

6.3 IVF or ICSI in Case of Non–Male Factor Infertility

ART treatments in the 1970s and 1980s consisted of conventional IVF to treat tubal factor infertility in combination with non–male factor infertility. Only after the introduction of ICSI in 1992, a tremendous decrease was noted in the use of conventional IVF to treat non–male factor infertility – with some centers performing almost exclusively ICSI, despite the lack of any evidence of a benefit of ICSI over conventional IVF (Figure 6.1). Couples with non–male factor infertility according to the WHO criteria (<1 $\times10^6$/mL round cells, concentration >15 $\times$ 10^6/mL, total motility >40 percent and progressive motility >32 percent; with a progressive motility >65 percent after capacitation, >4 percent normal morphology) (8), can easily undergo conventional IVF as the sperm velocity is sufficient for cumulus-zona penetration. On the other hand, in case of ICSI, rapidly progressive, morphologically normal sperm can be selected as well. This is translated into equal or improved fertilization rates and equal or improved blastocyst formation following conventional IVF. In case of negative selection during preimplantation development, this is attributed to the selection of abnormal sperm for ICSI which may result in low fertilization, abnormal cleavage, and developmental arrest. Also important, most prospective and retrospective studies have failed to demonstrate higher proportions of total fertilization failure after IVF.

These improved fertilization and developmental outcomes can be explained by the fact that conventional IVF facilitates a more "natural" selection of biologically fit sperm as compared to ICSI. During conventional IVF, the sperm is first exposed to the cumulus cells and it has been suggested that the cumulus has sperm chemotaxis properties, playing an important physiological role in the selection of functionally and genetically competent sperm. Different concerns have been raised – but not proven conclusively – regarding safety

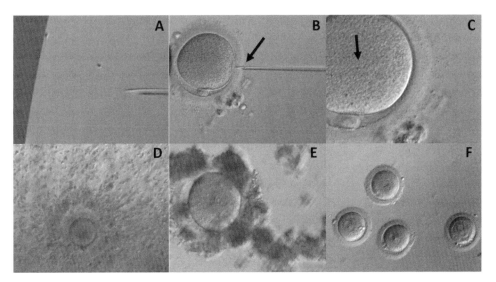

Figure 6.1 ICSI and conventional IVF. (A–C) Representation of ICSI and (D–F) conventional IVF. (A) Selection of the sperm for ICSI. (B) Position of the oocyte with the polar body at 6 o'clock and the injection needle with sperm (arrow) at 3 o'clock. (C) Mature oocyte after injection of the sperm (arrow) in the cytoplasm. (D) Cumulus oocyte complex after insemination with sperm on day 0 (sperm not visible). (E) Fertilized oocyte on day 1 with disintegrated cumulus. (F) Fertilized oocytes with a low number of spermatozoa attached to the zona pellucida.

of the ICSI technique, that also explain the absence of improved outcomes after ICSI: (1) the sperm is chosen based solely on the embryologists' subjective opinion of sperm phenotypic traits with no knowledge of the sperm genetic quality; (2) physical or biochemical disturbance of the ooplasm or the meiotic spindle; (3) errors in the selection of the injection site by inaccurate positioning of the injection needle with respect to the meiotic spindle; (4) the injection of biochemical contaminants; and (5) the injection of foreign sperm-associated exogenous DNA. Different selection methods have been tested to select the sperm with the highest fertilization potential for ICSI, like MACS or cumulus oocyte selected spermatozoa, however, in case of non–male factor infertility, conventional IVF allows the best selection of the most competent sperm.

Currently, the best treatment option in case of normozoospermia is conventional IVF, especially in patients undergoing their first ART treatment. To prevent total fertilization failure – be it after conventional IVF or after ICSI – in the first cycle, a split between IVF and ICSI can be recommended.

6.4 IVF or ICSI in Case of Male Factor Infertility

Male factor infertility is seen as an alteration in sperm concentration and/or motility and/or morphology in at least one of two sperm analyzes, collected 1 and 4 weeks apart. Sperm concentration, progressive motility, and morphology are all three key players in the success of IVF, with values below the reference limits having different impacts on the optimal treatment plan, conventional IVF or ICSI, for the infertile couple. Depending on the severity of the male factor, different treatment options should be applied; wrong treatment choice may lead to the complete failure of fertilization or the unnecessary use of ICSI. In general, patients with mild male factor infertility can mostly be treated with IVF and/or ICSI, while couples with severe male factor infertility can only be treated successfully with ICSI (Figure 6.2).

Treatment options for infertile men with a sperm concentration below the reference limit ($<15 \times 10^6$ per mL or $<39 \times 10^6$ per ejaculate) largely depend on the progressive motility and the volume of the ejaculate. The ESHRE guidelines for conventional IVF advise to use a progressively motile sperm concentration ranging between 0.1 and 0.5×10^6/mL (9). Patients with mild oligozoospermia in combination with high progressive motility have generally similar outcomes after conventional IVF and ICSI. On the other hand, patients with severe oligozoospermia might only benefit from ICSI, even if the sample is characterized by a high progressive motility. Interestingly, patients with severe oligozoospermia in combination with high posttesticular DNA fragmentation, have been shown to benefit from ICSI with testicular sperm compared to ejaculated sperm, as the sperm DNA fragmentation index appears to be lower in testicular sperm (10). Besides this, also higher pregnancy rates are observed with embryos generated from testicular sperm compared to ejaculated sperm.

Asthenozoospermia is characterized by an extremely low proportion of rapid progressive motility (<32 percent) in the fresh ejaculate. Treatment outcomes depend on the proportion of rapid (type A, <25 μm/s) versus slow (type B, 5–25 μm/s) progressively motile spermatozoa. As a specific velocity is required to penetrate the cumulus cells and the zona pellucida to obtain fertilization with conventional IVF, the absence or an extremely low proportion of rapid progressive spermatozoa is correlated with a high risk of very low fertilization or even total fertilization failure. Once fertilization is obtained, after conventional IVF or after ICSI, preimplantation development appears to be similar between both insemination methods. As the progressive motility is reduced, this coincides with an

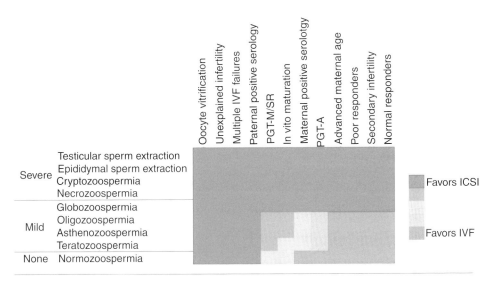

Figure 6.2 Indications for conventional IVF and ICSI. A black and white version of this figure will appear in some formats. For the colour version, please refer to the plate section.

increased proportion of immotile and/or dead spermatozoa in asthenozoospermic patients; prolonged exposure to dead spermatozoa in close vicinity of the oocyte, may lead to the production of reactive oxygen species and as such cause oxidative damage. The longer this exposure time, the higher the impact on further fertilization and embryo development. In case of a high concentration of immotile or dead spermatozoa, a short incubation IVF (three hours) is preferably used rather than conventional IVF with overnight exposure.

While abnormal sperm morphology has a deleterious effect on fertilization rates, patients with teratozoospermia (<4 percent normal morphology according to the strict Kruger criteria) may also benefit from conventional IVF, as it is thought that the zona pellucida provides a selective barrier for abnormally shaped spermatozoa. The reduced fertilization can be overcome by the use of high insemination concentration (HIC) for conventional IVF or by decreasing the medium volume to enhance the spatial interactions between gametes. However, once fertilized, development has been shown to be similar in IVF/ICSI sibling oocytes in patients with teratozoospermia, while ICSI development is adversely affected as abnormal sperm morphology increases. This is specially noted from day 3 of development, after the embryonic genome activation, when the paternal contribution is required, which is translated in increased developmental arrest to the blastocyst stage in ICSI embryos. If fertilization rates are improved in teratozoospermia after ICSI, they will be counterbalanced by superior blastocyst development after conventional IVF (11). A rare type of teratozoospermia, is globozoospermia (or round-headed sperm syndrome) accounting for <0.1 percent of male infertility. Mostly, these round-headed spermatozoa are lacking the acrosome and acrosomal enzymes, though some spermatozoa may have remnants of the acrosome. Acrosomeless spermatozoa are unable to penetrate through the zona and as such are unable to reach the oolemma. Conventional IVF will result in a total fertilization failure for patients with globozoospermia. The use of ICSI in combination with artificial oocyte activation is advised in infertile men with globozoospermia.

In nature, the absence of sperm movement is associated with sterility, as motility is the minimum necessity to penetrate the cervical mucus, move through the genital tract and penetrate the cumulus oocyte complex. Absence of motile sperm is a clear contra-indication for conventional IVF. It was only after the discovery of ICSI, that patients with azoospermia (no spermatozoa in the ejaculate), necrozoospermia (low percentage of live and high percentage of immotile spermatozoa in the ejaculate) and cryptozoospermia (spermatozoa absent from fresh preparations but observed in a centrifuged pellet) had the possibility to conceive a child. Whether the origin of azoospermia is immunological, genetic, obstructive, or non-obstructive, the standard treatment for these patients is ICSI. Even if motile sperm are found, the concentrations are too low to perform conventional IVF. Often, these patients are confronted with a high concentration of immotile sperm; the use of laser assisted immotile sperm selection, pentoxifylline, theophylline (Spermobil), or hypo-osmotic swelling test may serve as a useful indicator of sperm fertility potential.

6.5 Fertilization Failure

Shortly after the establishment of IVF, it became apparent that a high number of cycles, up to 40 percent, were affected by total fertilization failure (absence of any zygote presenting one female and one male pronucleus) or extremely low fertilization. As this outcome is emotionally devastating for the couple, it is critical to understand the etiology of this failure in order to advise subsequent successful treatment options. Though at increased risk for a repeated fertilization failure after IVF (30 percent), the fertilization capacity may differ between different stimulation cycles, suggesting that total fertilization failure cannot always be predicted. While the use of high insemination concentration (HIC) increases the fertilization potential for some patients, not all patients benefit from HIC. Urging for the development of different insemination techniques to increase fertilization potential, the use of ICSI has proven to be more beneficial in cycles with previous fertilization failures compared to HIC. The incidence of fertilization failure, be it after IVF or ICSI, is generally higher in cycles with lower oocyte yield. As the number of oocytes available increases, the risk of failure reduces tremendously (~1 percent). This negative correlation is also observed between the risk of fertilization failure and the number of mature oocytes. Naturally, at least one mature competent oocyte is required to obtain fertilization, not only nuclear maturity, but also cytoplasmic maturation.

Fertilization failure after conventional IVF is much lower in couples with non–male factor infertility (~10 percent) compared to couples with mild male factor infertility (45 percent). Despite using ICSI as the method of insemination, fertilization failure may still occur. A large retrospective study in Latin-America including almost 50,000 IVF or ICSI cycles in couples with non–male factor infertility, demonstrated a lower fertilization failure rate after conventional IVF (3.37 percent versus 4.49 percent) and this concurs with many other studies demonstrating equal or lower fertilization failure rates after conventional IVF with normozoospermia (12). However, the available evidence is conflicting as some older studies, albeit with limited patient numbers, have found a higher fertilization failure after IVF. The fact that some studies suggest that fertilization rates are higher with IVF in circumstances of normozoospermia may be attributed to the fact that ICSI oocytes are more prone to degeneration due to mechanical damage, which is not the case for oocytes inseminated by IVF. This damage may be induced during the denudation process as well as during the ICSI procedure itself. The enzymatic and mechanical stress during the removal of cumulus cells may cause a high degree of spindle deviations prior to the ICSI procedure; these are generally not observed after IVF, which allows a gentle and fast removal of the cumulus cells on day 1, especially if the oocyte is fertilized. During the ICSI procedure itself, mechanical damage to the oocyte may lead to degeneration, with operator variabilities showing up to 15 percent degeneration. While no further options are available after fertilization failure in ICSI oocytes, a rescue-ICSI procedure can be applied on day 1 on these failed-fertilized IVF oocytes; not only will this technique increase the fertilization rate for the patient, they also moderately increase pregnancy rates. On the other hand, persistent fertilization failures after conventional IVF, can mostly be solved with ICSI. Naturally they also depend on the competence of the oocyte, but increased fertilization and embryo development has been observed after ICSI in patients with fertilization failures from conventional IVF.

An important question is whether we are able to predict a total fertilization failure. Crucial here is to distinguish between failed oocyte activation due to sperm factor or the impaired ability of the oocyte to respond to the sperm. Asynchrony in the nuclear and cytoplasmic maturation of the oocyte may be responsible for the inability of the ooplasm to support decondensation of the sperm nucleus. While nuclear maturity can facilely be visualized by the extrusion of the first polar body, cytoplasmic maturation is not readily ascribable. For spermatozoa on the other hand, different tests are available to determine their competence to fertilize oocytes. The hamster ovum penetration test is an easy sperm function assay testing the capacity of human spermatozoa to fuse with zona pellucida-free golden hamster oocytes. As hamster oocytes may easily be activated by the injection procedure itself, alternatively, mouse oocytes can be injected with human sperm cells to test their ability to activate the oocyte in a mouse oocyte activation test. Another test is the hemizona assay in which two matching hemizona halves are allowed to bind sperm from a fertile control versus the test sample. Sperm DNA accelerated decondensation test, sperm DNA decondensation test, and sperm penetration assay can also be used to assess different aspects of sperm functionality and genomic integrity. However, with all these different screening tests available, every stimulation cycle and ejaculate being different, no test will give a 100 percent guarantee to prevent fertilization failure; not after conventional IVF and not after ICSI.

Assisted oocyte activation can be used to solve problems with persistent fertilization failure after ICSI, as spermatozoa are unable to induce the ooplasmic Ca^{2+} rise. Chemical stimulation with ionomycin, Ca^{2+}-ionophore and strontium chloride or even electrical stimuli are often used to activate human oocytes. Besides inconsistencies in fertilization outcomes, the Ca^{2+} oscillations induced by these agents do not always follow the physiological cascade, thereby questioning their effect on embryo development and even neonatal outcomes.

6.6 DNA Fragmentation

Sperm DNA fragmentation is damage in the sperm's DNA seen as breaks or separations in a single or double strand of the DNA. Spermatozoa with DNA damage are able to normally fertilize an oocyte and develop into a blastocyst-stage embryo. The human oocyte and embryos are equipped with mechanisms that can repair DNA damage, however, the ability of the oocyte or embryo to initiate repair is dependent on the cytoplasmic and genomic quality of the oocyte. The repair mechanisms are yet to be exploited but the undisputed fact is that DNA repair is impacted by increasing age.

DNA damage in the sperm can be induced by six mechanisms: (1) apoptosis during spermatogenesis; (2) DNA strand breaks during sperm chromatin remodeling; (3) post-testicular DNA fragmentation caused by oxygen radicals; (4) DNA fragmentation induced by endogenous caspases; (5) radiotherapy and chemotherapy; and (6) DNA damage induced by environmental toxicants, such as air pollution.

During spermatogenesis, 50–60 percent of germ cells are destined to be phagocytosed by Sertoli cells, these sperm cells exhibit an apoptotic marker such as Fas, p53, and phosphatidylserine. However, the process of apoptosis does not always operate efficiently leading to the presence of these defective sperm cells in the ejaculate.

Posttesticular sperm DNA fragmentation can be induced by many factors such as immature sperm that produce high levels of ROS, or oxygen radicals, and physiochemical factors such as temperature; these factors activate sperm caspases and endonucleases. It is worth mentioning that recent studies have shown that ejaculated sperm has higher DNA fragmentation levels than sperm from corpus and caput epididymis which is where the disulfide cross linking takes place (13).

6.7 Different Indications than Non–Male Factor Infertility

6.7.1 Female Infertility

Conventional IVF is an appropriate option for a young population with unexplained or tubal infertility with a normal response to ovarian stimulation. Though, for patients with unexplained infertility, the use of ICSI is sometimes encouraged to bypass potential fertilization barriers that could be the cause of the unexplained infertility.

The treatment of patients with an extremely low ovarian response is often challenging. The lower the number of oocytes retrieved, the higher the chances of total fertilization failure after conventional IVF, consequently, ICSI has gained popularity in patients with an extremely low number of oocytes retrieved. However, recent studies have shown that conventional IVF performs as good as ICSI in terms of fertilization capacity, embryo development, and improved live birth rates after conventional IVF, even in patients with only one oocyte retrieved. However, one important condition is the presence of normal sperm parameters.

The oocytes of woman with advanced maternal age have been assigned to have structural defects of the zona pellucida or cytoplasmic immaturity reducing the fertilization potential after conventional IVF. However, recent studies have explored the fertilization and developmental competence of woman with advanced maternal age and conventional IVF as well as ICSI perform equally well. Not unimportantly, similar results are obtained in poor ovarian response patients of advanced maternal age. Irrespective of female age, woman with poor oocyte quality (nuclear or cytoplasmic anomalies) or oocytes with repeated high degeneration rates after ICSI, may benefit from conventional IVF in case sperm parameters allow to do so.

6.7.2 Oocyte Vitrification

The most efficient way to fertilize cryopreserved oocytes is ICSI. Though conventional IVF has been sporadically explored after oocyte cryopreservation, the fertilization rates are extremely low. There are two main players determining the beneficial use of ICSI over IVF. First, oocytes are denuded before the cryopreservation procedure, as oocyte cryopreservation without cumulus cell removal has been shown to be far less efficient in terms of survival rate. Second, cryopreservation induces a cortical granule release, being highly apparent after slow freezing and less after vitrification. Both the absence of cumulus cells as the cortical granule release, diminish the fertilization capacity after conventional IVF.

6.7.3 In-Vitro Matured Oocytes

Early research on IVM with electron microscopy has shown mitochondrial degeneration, an increased apoptotic activity in the cumulus cells and a hardening effect of the zona pellucida, favoring the use of ICSI as a fertilization method (14). Conventional IVF has been applied on denuded oocytes with expected very low success rates; however, when conventional IVF is applied on the cumulus oocyte complex, similar fertilization rates can be obtained as compared to ICSI. As most clinics like to know the performance of their IVM system, ICIS is often opted as the method of choice to know the exact maturation rate. However, when nicely expanded cumulus complexes are available in combination with non–male factor infertility, conventional IVF can be applied.

6.7.4 Preimplantation Genetic Testing

In case of preimplantation genetic testing (PGT), the use of ICSI has been recommended by ASRM, SART, and ESHRE/PGDIS for all couples, even in case of non–male factor infertility. The motivation to choose ICSI over conventional IVF is to ensure monospermic fertilization, to eliminate potential paternal contamination from extraneous sperm attached to the zona pellucida or to prevent the presence of nondecondensed sperm within blastomeres or cumulus cells. Despite this suggestion, it has recently been shown that sperm DNA fails to amplify under the conditions used for trophectoderm (TE) biopsy samples, opening doors to the use of conventional IVF in PGT cycles, especially in non–male factor or mild male factor infertility. Aside from the adherence of sperm cells, genetic contamination of the trophectoderm (TE) samples from maternal cumulus cells, has also been suggested as possible factors adversely affecting the accuracy of genetic test results. Enzymatic removal of cumulus cells, combined with mechanical removal, is not always successful in removing all cumulus cells before ICSI, while mechanical pipetting of IVF oocytes prior to fertilization check allows a faster, easier, and less invasive removal of all cumulus cells.

The use of conventional IVF has been sporadically explored in PGT cycles in recent years. Similar euploidy rates were obtained for IVF and ICSI in PGT for monogenic disorders (PGT-M) on blastomeres; after fluorescent in situ hybridization (FISH) on blastomeres as well as after PGT for aneuploidies (PGT-A) on trophectoderm biopsies. However, the retrospective design of these studies, the absence of sperm parameters or significant differences in sperm concentration and motility between conventional IVF and ICSI, and the very limited information available after trophectoderm biopsy highlight the need for more in-depth analysis on the possible use of conventional IVF in PGT-A cycles.

6.7.5 Positive Serology

All assisted reproductive technologies (ART) involve handling of biological material and pose a potential hazard of transmitting diseases to personnel, to other patients' biological material and to the embryos resulting from the treatment. Male and female patients must be screened for infectious diseases such as Chlamydia trachomatis, hepatitis B virus (HBV), hepatitis C virus (HCV) and human immunodeficiency virus (HIV). Several ethical and medical considerations arise for treatment of patients with infectious samples, but the question in place is what will be the contribution of ICSI/IVF in the reduction of transmitting the disease to the offspring.

In cases where the female is infected with a transmitted disease, the method of choice for insemination will not contribute to the elimination or reduction of the disease or infection to the resulting embryos. While in cases where the male is infected (HBV, HIV, HCV), risk of transmission is reduced when ICSI is selected as the method of insemination, as the utilization of a single spermatozoon for insemination in conjunction with removal of the seminal fluid during sperm processing drastically reduces the chance of viral transmission (15).

6.7.6 Cryopreserved Sperm

Sperm cells cryopreservation involves the exposure of the sperm cells to cryoprotectants, followed by the gradual decrease of temperature below zero and finally the long-term storage in liquid nitrogen (−196°C). Sperm cells are easy to cryopreserve due to the tightly packed chromatin, low cytoplasmic volume, and the high surface to volume ratio, however cell damage can still occur for different reasons, such as; the formation of intracellular ice crystals and osmotic changes.

Sperm cryopreservation can cause negative impact on the sperm motility and viability, moreover, can cause structural changes in the acrosome, chromatin defects, and reduced mitochondrial activity (16). Although postthaw semen parameters are decreased compared to the fresh sample, this does not represent a limitation for ICSI since one viable sperm is required for each oocyte. Several studies have shown similar fertilization rate and embryo quality when using fresh sperm (ejaculate or testicular) compared to frozen sperm after ICSI (17). The same might not apply for conventional IVF, where fertilization rate might be compromised if sperm count and motility are impaired after thawing; however, embryo quality remains comparable with fresh ejaculate.

6.8 IVF versus ICSI Obstetric and Neonatal Outcomes

The health of children conceived through IVF/ICSI is of considerable interest. Several studies and meta-analyses have looked into the adverse outcome of ART babies, however, no affirmative conclusions are drawn. A wide range of challenges are encountered in obtaining and evaluating data from epidemiological studies, including small sample size, correction for confounding factors such as maternal age, incomplete reporting, and difficulty in defining the control population. Even without the addition of assisted human reproduction, there is increasing evidence that infertility or subfertility itself is an independent risk factor for obstetrical complications and adverse perinatal outcomes. An increased risk of congenital malformations is observed in ART children, even after adjustment for known confounders such as maternal age (18).

Risks of obstetric and perinatal morbidity such as hypertensive disorders of pregnancy, gestational diabetes, preterm delivery, and low birth weight have been associated with IVF. These adverse outcomes are largely due to an increased risk of multiple gestations in IVF, while these risks are reduced after single embryo transfer. The comparison of obstetric outcomes between conventional IVF and ICSI is not straightforward, as the adverse obstetric outcomes after ICSI are often related to the paternal infertility. However, two meta-analyses comparing the outcomes between IVF and ICSI were unable to find significant differences in birth defects between both insemination methods (19, 20).

Conventional IVF and ICSI are safe and successful treatments for infertility, these treatments are relatively new, and the data we have are limited to few decades. Well-controlled, large-scale, multicenter, prospective, long-term epidemiological studies are required to clearly identify the neonatal outcome of IVF/ICSI and naturally conceived children and the etiology behind it.

6.9 Cost of IVF versus ICSI

As the number of ART treatments are increasing worldwide, the increased use of ICSI and IVF has been associated with significant economic costs. Normally the decision of IVF treatment or ICSI treatment following an ovarian stimulation is dependent on the infertility factor as previously discussed. However, in cases where both treatment procedures are applicable, IVF provides generally a less expensive choice.

The cost of consumables used during an ICSI or IVF procedure do not differ significantly and are mostly limited to the use of specific injection needles and oocyte holding pipettes in ICSI procedure. But the main difference in cost is attributed to the specific equipment required to perform ICSI, maintenance, and labor-related costs. The intensity and specificity of ICSI procedure requires more careful training and qualification than that required for IVF.

References

1. Steptoe PC, Edwards RG. Birth after the reimplantation of a human embryo. Lancet 1978;2:366.

2. Hamori M, Stuckensen JA, Rumf D, et al. Zygote intrafallopian transfer (ZIFT): evaluation of 42 cases. Fertil Steril 1988;50(3):519–521.

3. Wikland M, Enk L, Hammarberg K, et al. Use of a vaginal transducer for oocyte retrieval in an IVF/ET program. J Clin Ultrasound 1987;15(4):245–251.

4. Malter HE, Cohen J. Partial zona dissection of the human oocyte: a nontraumatic method using micromanipulation to assist zona pellucida penetration. Fertil Steril 1989;51:139–148.

5. Palermo G, Joris H, Devroey P, et al. Induction of acrosome reaction in human spermatozoa used for subzonal insemination. Hum Reprod 1992;7:248–254.

6. Palermo G, Joris H, Devroey P, et al. Pregnancies after intracytoplasmic injection of single spermatozoon into an oocyte. Lancet 1992;340(8810):17–18.

7. Tesarik J, Greco E. The probability of abnormal preimplantation development can be predicted by a single static observation on pronuclear stage morphology. Hum Reprod 1999;14(5):1318–1323.

8. World Health Organization, Department of Reproductive Health and Research. WHO Laboratory Manual for the Examination and Processing of Human Semen. World Health Organization, 2010.

9. ESHRE Guideline Group on good practice in IVF labs. Revised Guidelines for Good Practice in IVF Laboratories. ESHRE, 2015.

10. Esteves SC, Roque M, Garrido N. Use of testicular sperm for intracytoplasmic sperm injection in men with high sperm DNA fragmentation: a SWOT analysis. Asian J Androl 2018;20(1):1–8.

11. Hotaling JM, Smith JF, Rosen M, et al. The relationship between isolated teratozoospermia and clinical pregnancy after in vitro fertilization with or without intracytoplasmic sperm injection: a systematic review and meta-analysis. Fertil Steril 2011;95(3):1141–1145.

12. Schwarze J, Jeria R, Crosby J, et al. Is there a reason to perform ICSI in the absence of male factor? Lessons from the Latin American Registry of ART. Hum Reprod Open 2017;2017:1–5.

13. Greco E, Scarselli F, Iacobelli M, et al. Efficient treatment of infertility due to sperm DNA damage by ICSI with testicular spermatozoa. Hum Reprod 2005;20 (1):226–230.

14. Hatirnaz S, Ata B, Hatirnaz ES, et al. Oocyte in vitro maturation: a systematic review. Turk J Obstet Gynecol 2018;15:112–125.

15. Wu MY, Ho HN. Cost and safety of assisted reproductive technologies for human immunodeficiency virus-1 discordant couples. World J Virol 2015;4:142–146.

16. Ozkavukcu S, Erdemli E, Isik A, et al. Effects of cryopreservation on sperm parameters and ultrastructural morphology of human spermatozoa. J Assist Reprod Genet 2008;25:403–411.

17. Kalsi J, Thum MY, Muneer A, et al. Analysis of the outcome of intracytoplasmic sperm injection using fresh or frozen sperm. BJU Int 2011;107:1124–1128.

18. Pinborg A, Henningsen AK, Malchau SS, et al. Congenital anomalies after assisted reproductive technology. Fertil Steril 2013;99(2):327–332.

19. Wen J, Jiang J, Ding C, et al. Birth defects in children conceived by in vitro fertilization and intracytoplasmic sperm injection: a meta-analysis. Fertil Steril 2012;97 (6):1331–1337.

20. Lie RT, Lyngstadaas A, Orstavik KH, et al. Birth defects in children conceived by ICSI compared with children conceived by other IVF-methods; a meta-analysis. Int J Epidemiol 2005;34(3):696–701.

Individualized Genetic Testing
Who Benefits?

Elpida Fragouli, Samer Alfarawati, and Anna Mantzouratou

7.1 Introduction

The main aim of preimplantation genetic testing (PGT), which up until recently was known as preimplantation genetic diagnosis (PGD), is the identification of embryos that are free of inherited genetic conditions. PGT can therefore be considered as a treatment option for couples where one or both partners are at risk of transmitting such a condition to their offspring. Inherited genetic conditions can affect gene function or chromosome structure, and could either be present in families or arise de novo. PGT for inherited mutations affecting gene function is defined as PGT for monogenic disorders or PGT-M, whereas PGT for inherited chromosome rearrangements is termed as PGT for structural rearrangements or PGT-SR (1). The selection and preferential transfer of healthy embryos could lead to the birth of babies who are free of the genetic disorder for which PGT was carried out, as well as potentially eradicate it from the family. Hence, PGT can be considered as an alternative form of prenatal diagnosis, with the added advantage that it avoids the termination of affected pregnancies.

The first PGT case took place over 20 years ago and involved the sexing of embryos with the use of the polymerase chain reaction (PCR) (2). During a PGT treatment cycle embryos are generated via in vitro fertilization (IVF), and sampled by employing a procedure called embryo biopsy. During biopsy one or more cells are removed from the embryo for subsequent genetic testing. Biopsy can take place at different stages of embryo development, as will be outlined further on. Embryo testing can occur with several different diagnostic strategies, depending on the type of condition for which PGT is being carried out.

A modified version of PGT termed PGT-A where the A stands for aneuploidy, aims to identify numerical chromosome abnormalities present in embryos. Soon after the development of methods capable of examining the chromosomes of embryos, in the context of PGT, it became evident that the presence of numerical abnormalities is extremely common during preimplantation development (e.g., 3, 4). The transfer of aneuploid embryos during IVF is unlikely to lead to ongoing pregnancies and live births. It has therefore been hypothesized that the preferential selection and transfer of chromosomally normal embryos would improve clinical outcomes for couples requiring IVF in order to conceive (5). Currently PGT-A is mostly used for couples going through IVF who are also considered to be at elevated risk of generating gametes and/or embryos affected by aneuploidy. Patient groups that would seek to use PGT-A to aid them achieve a pregnancy commonly include those who have experienced repeated implantation failure (RIF), or recurrent pregnancy loss (RPL), or where the female partner is of advanced reproductive age/advanced maternal age (ARA/AMA). PGT-A could also be used for male factor infertility cases where there is an indication of increased sperm aneuploidy, as well as for couples who have had previous aneuploid conceptions (1, 5, 6). The clinical procedures associated with PGT-A are very similar to those taking place during PGT, and will be outlined further on. A detailed overview of PGT-M, PGT-SR, and PGT-A will be undertaken in this chapter. Additionally, the clinical value, potential benefits, and drawbacks of genetic testing in the context of PGT-M, PGT-SR, and PGT-A will be discussed.

7.2 Embryo Sampling and Genetic Analysis

There are three different stages of early development during which embryo biopsy can take place, namely, before and after fertilization, on day 3 when the embryo is at the cleavage stage, or on days 5 or 6 when the embryo has undergone the first cellular differentiation into trophectoderm (TE, will give rise to the placenta), and inner cell mass (ICM, will give rise to the fetus) and has become a blastocyst (reviewed in 7). Biopsy taking place before and after fertilization involves the removal of the first and second polar bodies (PBs), respectively, cleavage-stage biopsy involves the removal of a single blastomere, whereas blastocyst-stage biopsy involves the removal of a few (usually three to five) TE cells. PB sampling can only be used for female carriers of genetic conditions as the analysis of these cells provides information on the status of the oocyte. Cleavage and blastocyst-stage sampling and analysis, on the other hand, provide information on the status of the embryo. Currently, blastocyst-stage biopsy is the most widely used and it is considered the least damaging to the embryo, as it samples cells from the TE that will form the placental tissue after implantation. PB biopsy is only employed in countries where embryo sampling is not allowed. Technical details for the three different biopsy stages, as well as their advantages and disadvantages, are summarized in Table 7.1.

A single cell contains 5–10 pg of DNA. The analysis of such minute DNA amounts during PGT, means that all diagnostic strategies will include an initial DNA amplification step, and can end up being technically demanding. Issues such as DNA contamination, amplification failure, or allele dropout (ADO) can all influence the diagnostic accuracy of PGT, especially when this takes place for the detection of mutations affecting gene function (PGT-M) (8). ADO is defined as the amplification failure of one of the alleles in a heterozygous cell. This amplification failure would cause the heterozygous cell to appear homozygous at the ADO affected locus, increasing in this way the misdiagnosis risk (4). To avoid such issues and maximize diagnostic accuracy, standard PGT-M approaches commonly use multiplex PCR methodologies, during which several different loci, including those affected by the mutation as well as others in the vicinity, are simultaneously amplified with the use of several distinct primer sets (9). The development of robust diagnostic PGT-M strategies requires careful protocol design optimization and validation, and can be lengthy and expensive. It is therefore not unusual for patients requesting PGT-M to have to wait for several months before starting their IVF cycle so as to undergo embryo testing. Moreover, PGT-M via multiplex PCR does not permit chromosome assessment, meaning that any aneuploid embryos will not be identified.

Recently an alternative PGT-M approach has been developed, termed karyomapping (10). Karyomapping employs an array platform which consists of approximately 300,000 single-nucleotide polymorphisms (SNPs). These SNPs are spread across the human genome, and during PGT-M are used to perform linkage analysis for the gene of interest and determine the presence of normal or mutated copies in the examined embryos (9, 10).

Table 7.1 Biopsy stages for preimplantation genetic testing

Biopsy type	When does it take place?	How does it take place?	Cell type removed	Type of errors assessed	Used for PGT-M, PGT-SR, and PGT-A?	Impact on embryo development?	Other considerations
First and second PBs	Sequentially on the oocyte retrieval day for first PB removal, and on day 1 after fertilization for second PB removal OR Simultaneously on day 1 after fertilization with removal of both first and second PBs	Acid Tyrode's, Mechanical, or Laser	Polar bodies which are by-products of oocyte meiosis I and II	Gene mutations or chromosome abnormalities of female origin	Yes	No	Compatible with fresh embryo transfer Biopsy process can be labor intensive Errors of male or postzygotic origin are not detected
Cleavage stage	Day 3 of preimplantation development	Acid Tyrode's, Mechanical, or Laser	Blastomere	Gene mutations of female and male origin Female and male meiotic and postfertilization mitotic chromosome abnormalities	Yes	Yes, cleavage-stage biopsy has been shown to reduce embryo implantation ability	Compatible with fresh embryo transfer Significant decrease of embryo mass at critical stage of preimplantation development

Table 7.1 (cont.)

Biopsy type	When does it take place?	How does it take place?	Cell type removed	Type of errors assessed	Used for PGT-M, PGT-SR, and PGT-A?	Impact on embryo development?	Other considerations
Blastocyst stage	Days 5 or 6 of preimplantation development	Mechanical, or Laser	Cells from trophectoderm part of the embryo which will form the placenta after implantation	Gene mutations of female and male origin Female and male meiotic and postfertilization mitotic chromosome abnormalities	Yes	Little if any	More cells available increasing diagnostic accuracy rates Trophectoderm and inner cell mass chromosome status may differ Not compatible with fresh embryo transfer Embryos may arrest before reaching blastocyst stage

Karyomapping enables the application of a single protocol for the PGT-M of several different inherited monogenic conditions, and importantly, allows the detection of certain types of chromosome abnormalities, such as losses leading to monosomies as well as some gains leading to trisomies. Additionally, the parental origin of meiotic chromosome errors can be determined.

Targeted next-generation sequencing (NGS) approaches have also been developed for PGT-M (11). NGS is a term that encompasses a variety of different methods capable of generating large quantities of DNA sequence information, rapidly, and at a low cost per base. Targeted NGS strategies have several advantages, over karyomapping, including the combination of accurate mutation detection, as well as all different aneuploidy types, and a potential decrease in costs associated with the procedure. A summary of the technical aspects, advantages, and limitations of the main PGT-M strategies can be found in Table 7.2.

For many years the main method for the PGT of chromosome abnormalities, both structural (PGT-SR) and numerical (PGT-A) was fluorescent in situ hybridization (FISH), with thousands of successful cycles having been carried out with its use. However, FISH-based PGT tests had several limitations. The most important of these limitations was the inability of FISH to assess the entire chromosome complement of biopsied samples. FISH PGT-SR or PGT-A strategies would only examine a limited number of chromosomes. Specifically, PGT-SR FISH protocols would focus on the chromosomes participating in the rearrangement, whereas those for PGT-A would target chromosomes that were most frequently seen in samples from spontaneous miscarriages and abnormal live births, and have been known to increase in malsegregation frequency with advancing female age, such as 13, 14, 15, 16, 18, 21, 22, and the sex chromosomes. Similar to PGT-M, most PGT-SR protocols had to be tailor-made for the structural rearrangement in question, and their optimization and validation could end up being technically challenging and lengthy. Moreover, FISH needed embryonic nuclei to be fixed on microscope slides, a process which required specialized skills and experience, and could lead to diagnostic problems, such as unclear or overlapping chromosome-specific probe signals.

The FISH associated shortcomings led to the development and use of new molecular comprehensive cytogenetic methodologies, which were capable of examining the entire chromosome complement of biopsied embryonic cells. The first molecular cytogenetic method to be used for the analysis of embryonic samples was metaphase comparative genomic hybridization (CGH) (e.g., 4). CGH involves a competitive hybridization of two differentially labeled DNAs, one which is normal (reference sample) and another one of unknown constitution (test sample) on a microscope metaphase slide, followed by analysis which will determine the karyotype of the test sample. Metaphase CGH evolved to microarray CGH (aCGH), a similar method which used microarray slides for the competitive hybridization to take place, rather than the metaphase ones (12). Other PGT-A approaches used SNP microarrays or fluorescent quantitative real-time PCR (13), whereas various different NGS strategies have been devised recently (14). NGS has several advantages, compared to other comprehensive chromosome screening approaches, and for this reason it has become the method of choice for both PGT-SR and PGT-A in recent years. Table 7.3 summarizes the technical details and compares each of the main PGT-A and PGT-SR diagnostic strategies.

Table 7.2 PGT-M diagnostic strategies

Methodology	Technical details	Work-up required?	Aneuploidy detection?	Other considerations
Multiplex PCR	Simultaneous amplification of mutation affected locus, and polymorphism in vicinity to detect contamination and ADO Several primer sets used Protocol design varies according to mutation	Yes	No, unless chromosome carrying the mutation is affected	Requires parental DNAs Test optimization could be complicated and lengthy Results available in time for fresh embryo transfer Recombination may affect diagnostic accuracy
Karyomapping	Array interrogating over 300,000 SNPs spread across human genome used Linkage analysis determines genetic status of embryo Universal protocol, irrespective of mutation in question	Yes, in cases where specific mutation detection is required	Yes	Requires parental DNAs and DNA from at least one affected relative Embryos must be frozen after biopsy, and unaffected ones can be transferred in subsequent cycle Possible issues with mutations arising de novo Recombination may affect diagnostic accuracy Issues with secondary findings, e.g., unaffected embryos which are aneuploid Issues with accurate identification of trisomies where 2 of the 3 chromosome copies are identical
Targeted next-generation sequencing	Encompasses a variety of different methods capable of generating large quantities of DNA sequence information, rapidly and at a low cost per base Primers for mutations used in addition to chromosome copy number assessment	Yes, to ensure that all primers combine without technical issues	Yes	Requires parental DNAs. Embryos must be frozen after biopsy, and unaffected ones can be transferred in subsequent cycle Recombination may affect diagnostic accuracy Issues with secondary findings, e.g., unaffected embryos which are aneuploid

Table 7.3 PGT-SR and PGT-A diagnostic strategies

Methodology	Technical details	Work-up required?	Aneuploidy types detected	Other considerations
FISH	Fluorescently labeled DNA probes used to target specific chromosome areas Multiple FISH rounds can be performed to increase number of chromosomes examined	Yes, for PGT-SR	Whole or segmental abnormalities for targeted chromosomes	Results available in time for fresh embryo transfer Unable to assess entire chromosome complement. Cell spreading on microscope slides may affect diagnostic accuracy FISH protocol efficiency and diagnostic accuracy may decrease with multiple FISH rounds
CGH	Competitive hybridization of differentially labeled DNA samples (DNA from the embryo sample: green; chromosomally normal reference DNA: red) to normal metaphase chromosomes on a microscope slide Ratio of green:red fluorescence along the length of each chromosome determines the relative number of chromosome copies in the test sample compared to the reference	No	Whole or segmental abnormalities for entire chromosome complement	Assesses entire chromosome complement Embryos must be frozen after biopsy, and normal ones can be transferred in subsequent cycle Labor intensive technically, requires expertise in both molecular genetic and cytogenetic methods Chromosome G-banding knowledge required for analysis

Table 7.3 (cont.)

Methodology	Technical details	Work-up required?	Aneuploidy types detected	Other considerations
aCGH	Competitive hybridization of differentially labeled DNA samples (DNA from the embryo sample: green; chromosomally normal reference DNA: red) to microarray slide spotted with DNA probes representing the entire length of all 24 chromosomes Ratio of green:red fluorescence on array DNA spots determines the relative number of chromosome copies in the test sample compared to the reference	No	Whole or segmental abnormalities for entire chromosome complement	Assesses entire chromosome complement Simpler fluorescence ratio evaluation, compared to CGH via automated analysis Shorter hybridization time compared to CGH Results available in time for fresh embryo transfer
SNP arrays	Analysis of large number (10,000–500,000) of SNPs found along the length of each of the 24 chromosomes via the use of an array platform Test and reference DNAs hybridized on separate areas of the array platform Embryo DNA sample is compared with parental DNAs to determine chromosome copy number and aneuploidy origin	No	Whole or segmental abnormalities for entire chromosome complement	Assesses entire chromosome complement Simpler cytogenetic evaluation, via automated analysis Embryos must be frozen after biopsy, and normal ones can be transferred in subsequent cycle

	Fluorescence intensity ratio between embryo DNA sample and reference sample also determines chromosome copy number		Whole abnormalities for entire chromosome complement	Assesses entire chromosome complement Simpler cytogenetic evaluation, via automated analysis Results available in time for fresh embryo transfer Unable to accurately detect abnormalities affecting segments of chromosomes
Q-PCR	Simultaneous amplification of a specific number of loci (usually 4) for each of the 24 chromosomes via fluorescence quantitative PCR Relative quantitation analysis of threshold cycle ($\Delta\Delta C_t$) determines chromosome copy number	No		
NGS	Embryo sample is amplified and then fragmented into pieces of 100–200 base pairs Sequencing of fragments follows Sequence data compared with reference genome and counted to determine chromosome copy number	No	Whole or segmental abnormalities for entire chromosome complement	Simpler cytogenetic evaluation, via automated analysis Embryos must be frozen after biopsy, and normal ones can be transferred in subsequent cycle Detection of mosaic chromosome abnormalities possible Issues with clinical management of mosaic diploid-aneuploid embryos

7.3 Preimplantation Genetic Testing for Inherited Disorders: Benefits and Considerations

Carriers of inherited genetic conditions that would seek PGT (M or SR) in order to achieve a pregnancy and a healthy live birth are usually fertile, unless their genetic condition affects their fertility. They are also generally reproductively younger, as far as female age is concerned. Therefore, the likelihood of a successful IVF-PGT cycle for this patient cohort is higher, compared to the PGT-A patient cohort.

PGT is generally considered as an ethically acceptable diagnostic pathway for most genetic disorders. However, questions have been raised by some for the use of PGT to detect mutations leading to late-onset diseases such as Huntington's, or to cancer predisposition such as BRCA1, BRCA2, neurofibromatosis 1 and 2, and Li Fraumeni (15), or more recently, for multifactorial conditions such as diabetes (16). As late-onset genetic conditions and gene mutations leading to cancer predisposition are associated with a significant negative impact on the carrier's quality and duration of life, the use of PGT should be an ethically acceptable option. PGT strategies for the diagnosis of multifactorial conditions, on the other hand, will require strict regulation, to ensure that they are not employed for the identification of nonpathogenic traits, such as eye color.

The clinical outcomes observed after the PGT of inherited genetic conditions have been assessed in several investigations. Konstantinidis et al. (9) performed PGT-M via karyo-mapping and conventional mutation analysis for 55 clinical cases and 35 different auto-somal dominant, autosomal recessive, X-linked, and incomplete penetrance disorders. Of the 251 blastocysts examined, karyomapping led to successful diagnosis of 250 (99.6 percent), and conventional mutation analysis strategies led to results for 243 (96.8 percent). The study reported on clinical outcomes for 20 of the 55 cases. Embryo transfers led to biochemical pregnancies for 18 couples (90 percent). Four (22 percent) of these pregnancies became early miscarriages and 14 (78 percent) were ongoing, 3 of which went to term at the time of writing this study.

The first births achieved after PGT-SR via the use of comprehensive chromosome screening methodologies, namely, CGH and aCGH were reported by Alfarawati et al. (17). The study described data on 20 cycles carried out for 16 couples. A pregnancy rate of 26.3 percent was observed for 19 of the 20 cycles. This lower pregnancy rate, compared to that reported by Konstantinidis et al. (9) in their PGT-M investigation, reflects the tendency that carriers of structural chromosome rearrangements have to generate a high proportion of aneuploid and/or unbalanced embryos, leading to a higher no transfer rate. One-third of the cycles reported by Alfarawati et al. (17) ended up being no transfers, due to the absence of euploid embryos. Conversely a 45.5 percent pregnancy rate per transfer was seen for cases having one or more chromosomally normal/balanced embryos.

Similar investigations using comprehensive chromosome screening approaches for the PGT-SR of a larger number of IVF cycles (18 for 75 IVF cycles, 19 for 74 IVF cycles) reported a clinical pregnancy rate of 61 percent, and a live birth rate of 52 percent per transfer and 38 percent per cycle (18, 19). The results of these investigations are summarized in Table 7.4.

What is interesting about data obtained via the use of molecular genetic approaches capable to assess the entire chromosome complement of cells biopsied from embryos for the purposes of PGT-M or PGT-SR, is the incidence of secondary findings. Secondary findings can be defined as findings identified during genetic testing which are unrelated to the

Table 7.4 Clinical outcomes after PGT-M and PGT-SR

Study	PGT type	Method used for PGT	No. of embryos analyzed	No. of cycles	Ongoing pregnancy rate per cycle
Konstantinidis et al. (2015)	PGT-M	Conventional mutation analysis and Karyomapping	251	55	78%
Alfarawati et al. (2011)	PGT-SR	CGH and aCGH	121	20	26%
Tobler et al. (2014)	PGT-SR	SNP arrays and aCGH	498	75	61%
Idowu et al. (2015)	PGT-SR	SNP arrays	539	74	38%

medical reason that the genetic testing is taking place for. Konstantinidis and colleagues (9) identified a total of 5 (2 percent) chromosomally abnormal blastocysts in the 250 embryos with PGT-M diagnosis. Monosomy, trisomy, and ploidy errors were detected via the use of karyomapping. Similarly, among 498 blastocysts undergoing PGT-SR via the use of SNP arrays or aCGH, 118 (24 percent) were characterized to be normal/balanced for the structural rearrangement, but were identified to be carrying unrelated chromosome errors (18).

Chromosome abnormalities of both meiotic and mitotic origin, are frequently observed during preimplantation development. Those of meiotic origin increase dramatically with advancing female age. Aneuploid embryos are unlikely to implant, if transferred, or if they do, have a high probability of miscarrying. Therefore, their identification during PGT-M or PGT-SR cycles, especially in cases of advanced female age, should lead to improved clinical outcomes. In other words, any pregnancies achieved would be free of the genetic condition and likely chromosomally normal. The flipside in all this is that the use of comprehensive molecular genetic approaches could lower the number of embryos available for transfer. The origin of these unrelated chromosome abnormalities is also important. If such errors are meiotic, then they will be present in all of the cells of the embryo, rendering it nonviable. If, on the other hand, these chromosome abnormalities arise postzygotically, and are present in only some of the embryonic cells, a phenomenon known as mosaicism, then the embryo's viability and implantation ability are likely to be reduced, but not completely absent making their clinical management problematic. This will be discussed further in a subsequent section. Results published to date suggest that the frequency of embryos with secondary findings is relatively low during PGT-M and PGT-SR. This means that any negative impact on the clinical outcomes during such cycles is likely to be minimal.

Couples where one or both of the partners are carriers of a genetic condition would most commonly turn to PGT after suffering multiple reproductive setbacks, including infertility, several miscarriages, or even the birth of children affected by the condition. PGT, if successful, will aid these couples to obtain healthy children. Hence, carriers of inherited conditions are bound to greatly benefit from genetic testing of their embryos.

7.4 Preimplantation Genetic Testing for Aneuploidy: Benefits and Considerations

The patient cohort that would consider PGT-A in order to achieve a clinical pregnancy and a healthy live birth, is somewhat different to the PGT-M and PGT-SR populations. Specifically, PGT-A would be considered in combination with IVF for couples with fertility issues. PGT-A indications include advanced female reproductive age (ARA), repeated unexplained implantation failure or miscarriages (RIF and RPL, respectively), male factor infertility (MF), or previous aneuploid conceptions with both partners having a normal karyotype. The main aim of PGT-A is to improve clinical outcomes after IVF, by decreasing the time to pregnancy, reducing miscarriage rates, and avoiding the transfer of aneuploid nonviable embryos. Currently, PGT-A is the most widely used PGT approach due to its relative simplicity and the ever-expanding patient groups who would request it.

As already mentioned, for many years PGT-A was performed via the use of FISH for the analysis of 5–12 chromosomes on blastomeres biopsied from cleavage-stage embryos. However, several randomized clinical trials (RCTs) demonstrated that this screening approach did not improve clinical outcomes after IVF (20). There were three main reasons for this failure: the inability of FISH to examine the entire chromosome complement of the biopsied cells, the high rate of chromosomal mosaicism during the cleavage stage of preimplantation development (21), and the negative impact the removal of a single blastomere had on the viability of the corresponding embryos (22).

The way that PGT-A was performed changed dramatically in the mid-2000s with the optimization of molecular cytogenetic methods capable of examining the entire chromosome complement of embryonic samples, and the improvement of IVF culture systems. This improvement meant that embryos could safely remain in culture until the final stage of preimplantation development, the blastocyst stage. Fragouli and colleagues (23) were the first to describe clinical data after the use of CGH for the cytogenetic analysis of TE samples biopsied from blastocyst-stage embryos. This cytogenetic analysis demonstrated that a significant number (62 percent) of blastocysts were euploid, but aneuploidy persisted to the final stage before implantation, and affected all chromosome groups. This and other similar investigations led to the development and clinical application of what has been characterized as PGT-A version 2 (v2). During PGT-A v2 molecular cytogenetic methods such as NGS are employed to assess the entire chromosome complement of a few cells biopsied from the TE part of the blastocyst-stage embryo. These molecular cytogenetic strategies usually yield results in a time frame which is longer to the period that an embryo can remain in culture. This means that all blastocysts are frozen by a procedure known as vitrification after TE biopsy. If any embryos are identified to have a normal chromosome complement after PGT-A, they can be thawed and prioritized for transfer in a subsequent cycle.

To date, several RCTs have been carried out to assess the clinical efficacy of PGT-A, and some had more promising results, than others. A meta-analysis report of some of these RCTs (24) suggested that PGT-A has the ability to improve clinical outcomes for a patient cohort with a normal ovarian reserve, although its usefulness was uncertain for poorer-prognosis groups. Two more recent RCTs came up with conflicting results. Specifically, Munné et al.

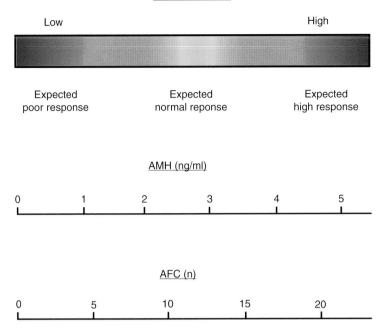

Figure 1.1 Ovarian reserve testing before the first IVF cycle would permit to categorize patients as expected poor, normal, or hyperresponders. The limits between low and normal response, and between normal and high response, are difficult to define accurately. Adequate dosage would maximize the success rate, minimizing the treatment burden or the OHSS risk. From La Marca et al. (12), with permission.

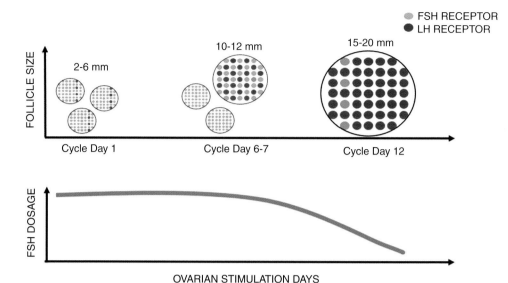

Figure 1.3 Follicle development and FSH/LH receptor expression during the ovarian stimulation. FSH receptors are predominant during the early follicular phase and have a steady reduction as the follicle increases in size and maturity (25). LH receptors are predominant at the late follicular phase. To reduce the incidence of progesterone elevation, the gonadotropin dose should be slowly reduced toward the late follicular phase, according to the patient's response, with no detrimental effect on follicle growth (21, 22).

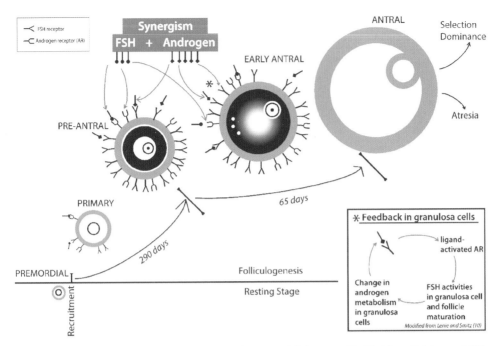

Figure 2.1 FSH and androgen receptors during small-growing follicle stages. Modified from Gleicher et al. (13), with permission.

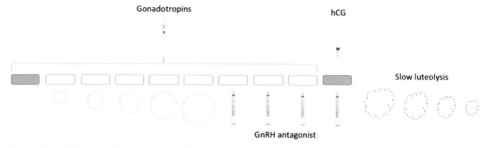

Figure 3.1 hCG trigger. Slow luteolysis offers an adequate luteal phase support.

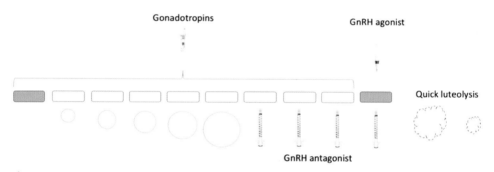

Figure 3.2 GnRHa trigger. Due to the quick luteolysis, additional drugs for luteal phase support are needed.

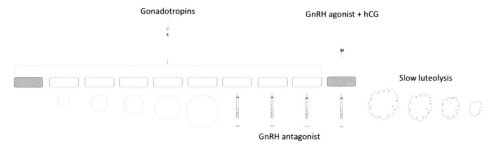

Figure 3.3 Dual trigger (GnRHa + hCG at the same time). Combines the advantage of reducing the risk of OHSS while maintaining an adequate luteal phase support and diminishing the incidence of EFS.

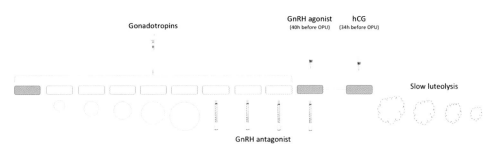

Figure 3.4 Double trigger (GnRHa at 40 hours before OPU + hCG at 34 hours before OPU). Follows the same principle as in the dual trigger strategy.

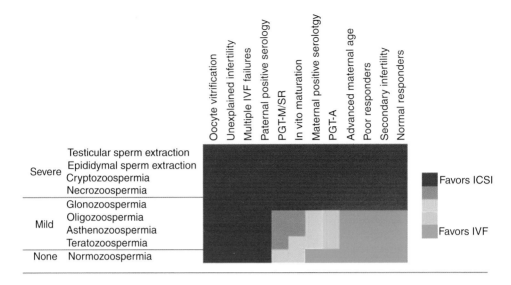

Figure 6.2 Indications for conventional IVF and ICSI.

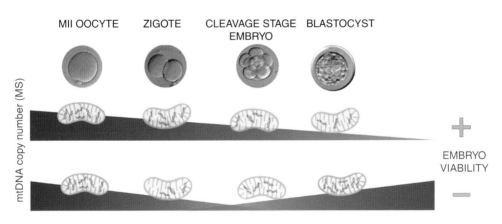

Figure 8.4 Relationship between embryo viability and mitochondrial DNA (mtDNA). The concentration of mtDNA is diluted among cells with each embryonic division, and this would be associated with better embryo quality. Adapted from Cecchino and García-Velasco (24).

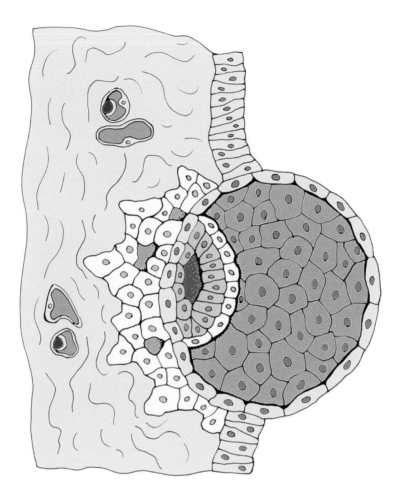

Figure 9.1 Diagrammatic representation of embryo implantation.

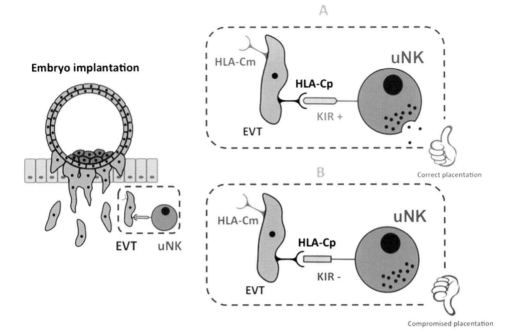

Figure 10.1 Maternal–fetal immune recognition in own oocytes single embryo transfer. (A) Correct activation through maternal KIR with a matched fetal HLA-C. (B) Inhibitory KIR signals after a contact with a mismatch fetal HLA-C.

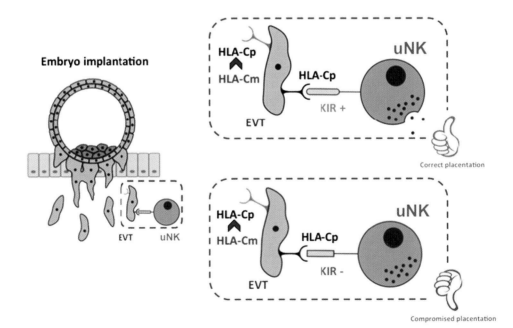

Figure 10.2 An egg donor embryo. The "maternal" HLA-C behaves as paternal, since, from a genetic point of view, it's foreign for the mother. So, in this case, the egg donor's HLA-C also needs to find the right receptor to induce good placentation.

(25) used NGS to examine TE samples biopsied from a patient group with a wide female age range (25–40 years), who were capable of generating at least two good-quality blastocysts, in a large multicenter RCT. The obtained results suggested that there may be some improvement in clinical outcomes for women of advanced reproductive age. Conversely, Verpoest and colleagues (26) in their multicenter RCT did not show a difference in clinical pregnancy rates between their test and control patient groups, irrespective of female age. It should be noted, however, that this RCT took place via first and second PB biopsy followed by aCGH analysis, and this strategy is generally not commonly used for PGT-A.

Skeptics of PGT-A argue that this procedure may damage and/or exclude viable embryos from transfer. There are two main issues with the way that PGT-A is being carried out currently: the first one is the biopsy procedure. Irrespective of the developmental stage during which the biopsy takes place, it requires a lengthy training period for the embryologists performing it to ensure that the viability of an embryo is not compromised, and the purchase of expensive laser equipment. Moreover, the biopsy procedure itself is not standardized, with different embryologists removing varying numbers of TE cells from blastocysts. It is likely, that removal of more than five TE cells will have an adverse impact on the viability and implantation ability of an embryo. The second issue is a biological phenomenon known as mosaicism.

Mosaicism can be defined as the presence of two or more chromosomally distinct cell lines in the same embryo. Mosaicism arises from chromosome malsegregation taking place during the mitotic divisions after fertilization, and leads to the formation of three different embryo types:

1. Mosaic diploid-aneuploid: these embryos consist of a combination of normal and chromosomally abnormal cells.
2. Mosaic aneuploid: these embryos consist of a combination of chromosomally abnormal cells, with one or two chromosomes being affected.
3. Chaotic: these embryos consist of a combination of chromosomally abnormal cells, with multiple chromosomes being affected.

The presence of mosaic chromosome abnormalities in preimplantation embryos has been known for years (21). Aneuploidy of mitotic origin and the resulting mosaicism became more clinically relevant recently due to the increasing use of NGS for the purposes of PGT-A. NGS is a much more sensitive method, compared to, e.g., aCGH. Therefore, in addition to chromosome errors present in all of the TE cells, NGS is capable of identifying aneuploidies present in some of the biopsied TE cells. The detection of mosaic chromosome abnormalities has had a negative impact on PGT-A's diagnostic accuracy, and it has caused confusion about which is the best way to clinically manage embryos that consist of a combination of normal and aneuploid cells, in other words, those characterized as mosaic diploid-aneuploid.

Several studies have examined the viability and implantation ability of mosaic diploid-aneuploid embryos, and the findings of these are summarized in Table 7.5 (27–30). Data from these studies clearly show that mosaic diploid-aneuploid blastocysts are associated with significantly lower implantation and pregnancy rates, compared to completely euploid embryos, and higher miscarriage rates. These investigations formed the basis of a group of guidelines providing advice on the clinical management of blastocyst-stage embryos with

Table 7.5 Clinical outcomes after the transfer of mosaic diploid-aneuploid blastocysts

Study	No. of mosaic embryos	No. of chromosomally normal embryos	Implantation rate for mosaic embryos	Implantation rate for chromosomally normal embryos	Miscarriage rate for mosaic embryos	Miscarriage rate for chromosomally normal embryos	Pregnancy rate for mosaic embryos	Pregnancy rate for chromosomally normal embryos
Greco et al. (2015)	18	-	44%	-	11%	-	33%	-
Fragouli et al. (2017)	44	51	30%	56%	56%	17%	15%	46%
Munné et al. (2017)	143	1,045	53%	71%	24%	10%	41%	63%
Spinella et al. (2018)	78	251	38%	55%	8%	8%	30%	47%

different types of PGT-A results, which were recently published by the International Society of Preimplantation Genetic Diagnosis (PGDIS) (31). Briefly, these guidelines are as follows:

1. If any chromosomally normal embryos are identified during PGT-A, then they should be prioritized for transfer.
2. Embryos with chromosome abnormalities present in all of the cells of the TE biopsy should not be considered for transfer during PGT-A.
3. Mosaic embryos may be considered for transfer in the absence of chromosomally normal embryos, and if another IVF cycle with PGT-A is unlikely, if, e.g., the female patient is of advanced reproductive age.
4. Embryos characterized as low-level mosaics, in other words, those with the mitotic chromosome abnormality present in a minority of the biopsied TE sample, should be prioritized for transfer over those characterized as high-level mosaic having the chromosome abnormality present in the majority of the TE sample.
5. Prioritization of mosaic embryos for transfer should also be based on the number of errors present, and which chromosomes are affected.
6. Patients considering the transfer of a mosaic embryo should have a detailed discussion with a genetic counselor, in order to understand all risks associated with such a transfer.
7. If a pregnancy is established after the transfer of a mosaic embryo, then the couple should be advised to have a prenatal test preferably via amniocentesis to ensure the resulting fetus is free of any chromosome errors.

Unlike couples seeking PGT for an inherited genetic condition who are almost always fertile, patients requesting PGT-A generally have a complicated and sometimes very poor reproductive history. Studies published to date, including some RCTs, suggest that PGT-A could be of benefit for women with normal ovarian reserve, as well as for women of advanced reproductive age. It is unclear, however, if PGT-A would be useful for other indications. More well-designed and executed multicenter RCTs, and a better stratification of indications are necessary to determine with certainty if PGT-A is of benefit for the patient groups requesting it, in order to aid them achieve a pregnancy followed by a healthy live birth.

7.5 Conclusions

To summarize, there are two approaches for embryo testing, PGT (M or SR) and PGT-A. The patient groups who would consider these as a means for achieving a clinical pregnancy followed by the birth of a healthy baby are very different. Patients requesting PGT-M or PGT-SR are in most cases fertile, but they are carriers of gene mutations or chromosome rearrangements which lead to inherited genetic diseases, miscarriages, or the birth of children with congenital or mental disabilities. PGT-A patients, on the other hand, are a more diverse group, and in their vast majority have difficulty conceiving naturally. It is widely accepted that PGT-M and PGT-SR are capable of assisting the patient groups requesting them in having healthy children. Conversely, the clinical benefit of PGT-A remains unclear, to date at least. Several RCTs have demonstrated an improvement in implantation and pregnancy rates for certain patient groups, but these benefits are not universal.

Questions have been raised about the safety and diagnostic accuracy of PGT, due to the detection of secondary findings when employing diagnostic methodologies capable of examining the entire genome of biopsied embryonic samples. The appropriate stratification of indications, and collection of information on PGT methodology, and the health of children born as a result of such approaches are critically important. The efficacy and clinical benefit of PGT-A, in particular, need to be further investigated in well-designed multicenter prospective RCTs.

References

1. Harper JC, Aittomäki K, Borry P, et al. Recent developments in genetics and medically assisted reproduction: from research to clinical applications. Eur J Hum Genet 2018;26:12–33.

2. Handyside AH, Kontogianni EH, Hardy K, et al. Pregnancies from biopsied human preimplantation embryos sexed by Y-specific DNA amplification. Nature 1990;344:768–770.

3. Delhanty JD, Harper JC, Ao A, et al. Multicolour FISH detects frequent chromosomal mosaicism and chaotic division in normal preimplantation embryos from fertile patients. Hum Genet 1997;99:755–760.

4. Wells D, Delhanty JD. Comprehensive chromosomal analysis of human preimplantation embryos using whole genome amplification and single cell comparative genomic hybridization. Mol Hum Reprod 2000;6:1055–1062.

5. Geraedts J, Sermon K. Preimplantation genetic screening 2.0: the theory. Mol Hum Reprod 2016;22:839–844.

6. Munné S, Lee A, Rosenwaks Z, et al. Diagnosis of major chromosome aneuploidies in human preimplantation embryos. Hum Reprod 1993;8:2185–2191.

7. Cimadomo D, Capalbo A, Ubaldi FM, et al. The impact of biopsy on human embryo developmental potential during preimplantation genetic diagnosis. Biomed Res Int 2016;2016:7193075.

8. Thornhill AR, Snow K. Molecular diagnostics in preimplantation genetic diagnosis. J Mol Diagn 2002;4:11–29.

9. Konstantinidis M, Prates R, Goodall NN, et al. Live births following Karyomapping of human blastocysts: experience from clinical application of the method. Reprod Biomed Online 2015;3:394–403.

10. Natesan SA, Bladon AJ, Coskun S, et al. Genome-wide karyomapping accurately identifies the inheritance of single-gene defects in human preimplantation embryos in vitro. Genet Med 2014;16:838–845.

11. Treff NR, Forman EJ, Scott RT Jr. Next-generation sequencing for preimplantation genetic diagnosis. Fertil Steril 2013;99: e17–e18.

12. Fragouli E, Alfarawati S, Spath K, et al. The origin and impact of embryonic aneuploidy. Hum Genet 2013;132:1001–1013.

13. Northrop LE, Treff NR, Levy B, et al. SNP microarray based 24 chromosome aneuploidy screening demonstrates that cleavage-stage FISH poorly predicts aneuploidy in embryos that develop to morphologically normal blastocysts. Mol Hum Reprod 2010;16:590–600.

14. Wells D, Kaur K, Grifo J, et al. Clinical utilization of a rapid low-pass whole genome sequencing technique for the diagnosis of aneuploidy in human embryos prior to implantation. J Med Genet 2014;51:553–562.

15. Sermon K, Van Steirteghem A, Liebaers I. Preimplantation genetic diagnosis. Lancet 2004;363:1633–1641.

16. Treff NR, Zimmerman R, Bechor E, et al. Validation of concurrent preimplantation genetic testing for polygenic and monogenic disorders, structural rearrangements, and whole and segmental chromosome aneuploidy with a single universal platform. Eur J Med Genet 2019;62:103647.

17. Alfarawati S, Fragouli E, Colls P, et al. First births after preimplantation genetic diagnosis of structural chromosome abnormalities using comparative genomic hybridization and microarray analysis. Hum Reprod 2011;26:1560–1574.

18. Tobler KJ, Brezina PR, Benner AT, et al. Two different microarray technologies for preimplantation genetic diagnosis and screening, due to reciprocal translocation imbalances, demonstrate equivalent euploidy and clinical pregnancy rates. J Assist Reprod Genet 2014;31:843–850.

19. Idowu D, Merrion K, Wemmer N, et al. Pregnancy outcomes following 24-chromosome preimplantation genetic diagnosis in couples with balanced reciprocal or Robertsonian translocations. Fertil Steril 2015;103:1037–1042.

20. Mastenbroek S, Twisk M, Veen F, et al. Preimplantation genetic screening: a systematic review and meta-analysis of RCTs. Hum Reprod Update 2011;17:454–466.

21. Wells D, Delhanty JD. Comprehensive chromosomal analysis of human preimplantation embryos using whole genome amplification and single cell comparative genomic hybridization. Mol Hum Reprod 2000;6:1055–1062.

22. Scott RT, Upham KM, Forman EJ, et al. Cleavage-stage biopsy significantly impairs human embryonic implantation potential while blastocyst biopsy does not: a randomized and paired clinical trial. Fertil Steril 2013;100:624–630.

23. Fragouli E, Lenzi M, Ross R, et al. Comprehensive molecular cytogenetic analysis of the human blastocyst stage. Hum Reprod 2008;23:2596–2608.

24. Dahdouh EM, Balayla J, García Velasco JA. Comprehensive chromosome screening improves embryo selection: a metaanalysis. Fertil Steril 2015;104:1503–1512.

25. Munné S, Kaplan B, Frattarelli J, et al. Global multicenter randomized controlled trial comparing single embryo transfer with embryo selected by preimplantation genetic screening using next-generation sequencing versus morphologic assessment. Fert Steril 2017;108:e19.

26. Verpoest W, Staessen C, Bossuyt PM, et al. Preimplantation genetic testing for aneuploidy by microarray analysis of polar bodies in advanced maternal age: a randomized clinical trial. Hum Reprod 2018;33:1767–1776.

27. Greco E, Minasi MG, Fiorentino F. Healthy babies after intrauterine transfer of mosaic aneuploid blastocysts. N Engl J Med 2015;373:2089–2090.

28. Fragouli E, Alfarawati S, Spath K, et al. Analysis of implantation and ongoing pregnancy rates following the transfer of mosaic diploid-aneuploid blastocysts. Hum Genet 2017;136:805–819.

29. Munné S, Blazek J, Large M, et al. Detailed investigation into the cytogenetic constitution and pregnancy outcome of replacing mosaic blastocysts detected with the use of high-resolution next-generation sequencing. Fertil Steril 2017;108:62–71.

30. Spinella F, Fiorentino F, Biricik A, et al. Extent of chromosomal mosaicism influences the clinical outcome of in vitro fertilization treatments. Fertil Steril 2018;109:77–83.

31. Cram DS, Leigh D, Handyside A, et al. PGDIS position statement on the transfer of mosaic embryos. RBM Online 2019;39 e1–e4.

Chapter

Individualized Embryo Selection

Irene Hervás, Lucía Alegre, Lorena Bori, and Marcos
Meseguer

8.1 Introduction

It is 40 years since the birth of the first baby conceived through in vitro fertilization (IVF).
From then on, remarkable progress has been made in the management of infertility and
assisted reproductive technology (ART). The improvements in clinical practice, such as
ovarian stimulation protocols, embryo culture conditions, and vitrification protocols, have
led to improved success rates globally.

One of the most important changes that transformed routine work in the IVF laboratory
was the extended culture-to-blastocyst stage (corresponding to day 5 [D5] or day 6 [D6] of
embryonic development). The study of the nutritional requirements of human embryos at
different stages of development led to the development of stage-specific culture (sequential
media), allowing embryo development beyond cleavage stage. With the use of sequential
media, blastocyst development rates are as high as 60 percent (1).

A major advance was the creation of single-step media that permits prolonged continued embryo culture to D5 stage, providing all the nutrients throughout the embryonic
development. These are the media used in the most recent generation of incubators with
time-lapse technology, which have the advantage that embryos are not disturbed.

Embryos with developmental potential that undergo genome activation at morula stage
are capable of reaching blastocyst stage. Furthermore, extended culture-to-blastocyst stage
enables the selection of the most competitive embryo for transfer. On this basis, the majority
of embryo transfers are now performed at blastocyst stage instead of cleavage stage (2).

8.2 Extended Culture and Blastocyst-Stage Transfer:
Advantages and Disadvantages

Embryo transfer at D5 presents advantages over the traditional cleavage-stage transfer.
First, extended culture-to-blastocyst stage enables a proper assessment of embryo quality
and viability, allowing better embryo selection prior to transfer. Second, the blastocyst is the
stage when the embryo reaches the uterus in natural conception, whereas transfer in
cleavage stage is not in synchrony with the maternal endometrium. That may cause stress
and reduce implantation potential. Ultimately, previous studies have reported that blastocyst embryos have higher implantation rates and, consequently, increased pregnancy and
live birth rates in good-prognosis patient (2, 3).

Extended embryo culture allows the examination of embryos at a more advanced stage
of development, which makes embryo selection more accurate. The selection of the best
embryo to transfer is based on the morphological assessment during the first development

stages and in the final blastocyst stage. Embryo evaluation routine is normally performed by a series of single observations, by light microscopy, at set times. In fact, there is general consensus only for embryo morphology appraisal (4).

Traditional morphological evaluation of embryos examines the embryo at certain stages of development. On D3 the cleavage-stage embryos are assessed to observe the cell number, cellular symmetry and size, fragmentation score, and multinucleation, which is an estimation of embryo quality; however, their developmental potential to arrive at blastocyst stage is not determined. On D5 the embryo quality is assessed by evaluating the stage of development and the inner cell mass (ICM) and the trophectoderm (TE) of all blastocysts (4).

The Istanbul consensus established a scale-scoring system for blastocyst-stage embryos considering the stage of development and the aspect of ICM and TE, 1 being the best embryo and 4 the worst, as a common guide for embryologists around the world (4). The selection of the embryo with the best morphology for transfer is related to the implantation potential and pregnancy success, which depends on the embryo quality (5).

Nonetheless, embryo culture-to-blastocyst stage also has disadvantages. When the embryonic culture is lengthened until D5 or D6, the number of embryos that get to this stage is declining, so the risk of couples of not having embryos available for transfer (higher rate of cancelled cycles) is increased or they have fewer embryos available for cryopreservation (3).

Several studies confirmed that pregnancies, resulting from blastocyst transfer were associated with a higher relative risk of preterm and very preterm delivery and an increased likelihood of monozygotic twins and congenital anomalies compared with transfer of cleavage stage. Other groups have shown an altered sex ratio in blastocyst stage and epigenetic modifications in blastocyst cells due to extended culture which could affect the future offspring (2).

It is important to note that not all embryologist advocate blastocyst-stage transfer but that the stage of embryos to be transferred should be adapted to both the woman's characteristics and her previous IVF treatments, if any. The most recent Cochrane meta-analysis (including 27 RCTs) showed mixed findings. There was evidence that cleavage-stage transfers were associated with higher cumulative clinical pregnancy rates than blastocyst-stage fresh transfers. By contrast, a moderate higher live birth rates with blastocyst transfer per couple was found. There were no differences between the groups in multiple pregnancy rates or miscarriage (1).

However, all the studies included in this review are heterogeneous in design and protocols, which constitutes an important bias for the analysis. Future RCTs should report the clinical outcomes rates to help embryologists and patients undergoing ART choose the best treatment option available (1).

8.3 MET versus SET

The increase of knowledge of embryonic development has initiated changes not only in the embryo transfer timing, but also in the number of embryos to transfer. Since the beginning of ART, the most widespread strategy included multiple embryo transfer (MET) to increase the chance of pregnancy.

The problems associated with multiple pregnancies (twins or pregnancies of higher order) are well known for both the mother and the fetuses, with increased maternal morbidity and perinatal complications. Preterm labor, hypertension, preeclampsia, and a cesarean delivery are some of the known medical complications for the mother. In addition, neonatal complications such as low birthweight, neurological damage, respiratory distress, and even perinatal mortality are strong arguments in favor of reducing multiple pregnancies (6).

In addition, multiple births are associated with an increased incidence of familiar stress, anxiety, and depression. Medical assistance for these women is more complicated throughout pregnancy owing to the antenatal, obstetric, and neonatal complications, which is reflected in an increase of the economic burden to society and families (7, 8).

In order to avoid the problems associated with multiple pregnancies, a single embryo transfer (SET) policy should be encouraged worldwide (Table 8.1). Nowadays, the global trend is to reduce the number of embryos transferred in favor of SET (6).

The European Society of Human Reproduction and Embryology (ESHRE) has been collecting all national IVF data of European countries since 1997. Within the most recently published registers, in both IVF and ICSI cycles: 31.4 percent were SET [34.9 percent in 2014]; 54.5 percent were two embryos transfer (56.3 percent in 2013); and 10.6 percent were three or more embryos transfer (11.5 percent in 2013) (Figure 8.1). This evolution resulted in 82.5 percent of singleton births, 17.0 percent twins, and 0.5 percent triplets (10).

The Human Fertilisation and Embryology Authority defined IVF success as the birth of a healthy, term child with normal weight, not achieving a pregnancy. Furthermore, they established a strategy to reduce multiple pregnancy rates (MPR) below 10 percent in the UK clinics. To date, 86 percent of UK IVF clinics have achieved an average MPR of 11 percent (6).

Other countries have similar policies to limit the number of embryos transferred: Hungary, India, Italy, and Spain limit the number of embryos that can be transferred to three; France and Japan limit to two embryos; Turkey, Sweden and Belgium require SET for most transfers; and in Australia, in 2013 SET was performed in 78.9 percent of all IVF cycles (6, 8).

The American Society for Reproductive Medicine (ASRM) published a clinical guideline recommending the number of embryos to be transferred in IVF cycles, depending on the mother's age and the donor eggs' age in oocyte donation program, but those guidelines do not have the force of law (11).

The shift toward SET to avoid medical complications has coincided with the extended culture-to-blastocyst stage and improvements in embryo selection; however, some embryo transfers are still performed at the cleavage-stage at D3. Recent reviews addressed this issue, comparing the clinical outcomes rates of SET or DET in both embryo-stages, cleavage, and blastocyst (1, 6–9).

In clinical practice, it is important to decrease the risk of multiple pregnancies, while maximizing their chance of live birth. When an SET policy is considered, it is important to take into account the age of the female partner; her gynecological, obstetric, and medical history; her ovarian reserve; previous IVF treatments; the number of embryos per cycle and their quality; and the number of embryos available for transfer. As a global policy about when to perform SET or MET does not exist, only recommendations for clinical practice can be given (9).

The Cochrane review assessing this issue showed different conclusions (7). There was no evidence of a significant difference in cumulative birth rates when compared with a single DET cycle with a repeat SET at cleavage-stage (either two fresh cycles or a fresh plus frozen cycle) (42 percent vs. 31–44 percent, respectively). By contrast, the MPR was lower in repeated SET (0–2 percent instead of 13 percent with DET). When a single SET versus

Table 8.1 Embryo transfer policies in different countries

Country	Legislation
Australia	No legislation; SET advised <35 on first fresh cycle; no more than 2 advice <40
Austria	Legislation restricts the number of eggs which can be used in IVF. All fertilized embryos must be transferred
Belgium	Legislation; <36 first cycle must have SET
Canada	No legislation only guidelines suggesting SET in patient <35 years in a first or second cycle and consider SET in patients 36 and 37 with good prognosis Quebec introduced legislation in 2010 which states every cycle should be SET unless there are suboptimal conditions and clinical justification is given
Denmark	No legislation
Estonia	<3 embryos can be transferred
Finland	No legislation
France	Restricted to DET; if more than 2, clinical justification required
Germany	Legislation restricts the number of eggs which can be used in IVF; all fertilized embryos must be transferred
Greece	No legislation; recommended >3 embryos transferred for women up to age of 40 and up to 4 >40
Hungary	State regulation limits the number to transfer to >3 except in exceptional circumstances when up to 4 can be transferred
India	Guidelines: max of 3 embryos can be transferred
Italy	Law restricts number of eggs which can be fertilized; all resulting embryos must be replaced
Japan	Recommendation by Japanese Society of Obs and Gynae; max 2 embryos since 2008
Luxemburg	No legislation
Netherlands	No legislation
New Zealand	Guidance related to funding: if publicly funded <35, first or second cycle SET; ≤2 embryos (fresh or frozen) <40
Norway	No legislation
Portugal	Law contains general addict that MET should be avoided if possible
Spain	Legislation in 2006; max 3 embryos can be transferred
Sweden	State legislation states in principle only 1 embryo should be replaced apart from in exceptional circumstances
Switzerland	Legislation restricts the number of eggs which can be used in IVF; all fertilized embryos must be transferred
Turkey	Legislation in March 2010 favoring SET-limits <35 to SET and >35 to DET

Table 8.1 (cont.)

Country	Legislation
USA	No overall legislation. Guidelines suggest SET should be offered to patients <35, no more than 2 embryos should be transferred; patients 37–39, no more than 2 cleavage embryos in favorable prognosis patients or if blastocyst transfer; if using cleavage-stage transfer in poor prognosis ≥3 embryos should be replaced; no more than 3 embryos cleavage or 2 blastocyst in patients 38–40 years with favorable prognosis; other patients in this group ≥4 cleavage embryos or ≥3 blastocyst transferred; in patients 41–42 no more than 5 cleavage-stage embryos or 3 blastocysts; in patients with 2 or more previous failed cycles one additional embryo can be transferred in each category No limit on patients >43 years old In donor cycles, if the donor is <35, SET should be strongly recommended

Note. eSET, elective single embryo transfer; DET, double embryo transfer.
Source: Adapted from Harbottle et al. (9).

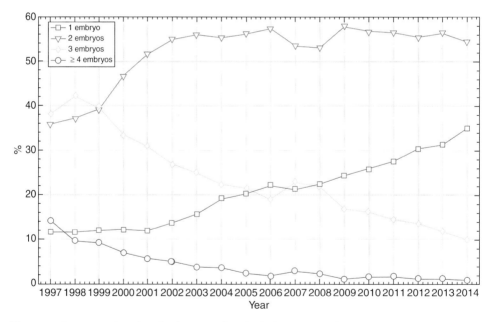

Figure 8.1 Proportion of number of embryos transferred in fresh IVF + ICSI cycles in Europe (1997–2014). Adapted from De Geyter et al. (10).

single DET was evaluated (both in cleavage and blastocyst stage), the live birth rate was significant lower in SET cycles compared with DET cycles (24–33 percent and 45 percent, respectively). Also, the MRP was significantly lower with SET (1–3 percent vs. 14 percent in

DET cycles). Nonetheless, studies comparing cleavage stage with blastocyst-stage transfers were excluded.

Most of the evidence currently available is derived from patients with a good prognosis, defining the SET strategy as the best option for women who undergo ART. Future studies should include patients with poor prognosis (older age, lack of good-quality embryos, previous failed IVF) (6). In addition, more RCTs comparing single or multiple blastocyst-stage transfer are necessary due to the lack of them, in order to establish a proper reproductive strategy.

Single embryo transfer is the best strategy to reduce multiple pregnancies but this needs to be balanced against the risk of compromising the overall pregnancy and live birth rates. The aim should be to enhance individualized embryo selection at the blastocyst stage in line with the existing clinical parameters, achieving a higher implantation potential, and to improve cumulative live birth rates.

8.4 Individualized Embryo Selection

In routine clinical practice, embryo transfer is the final step in an IVF cycle. Several parameters such as embryo quality, embryo selection, uterine receptivity, and the embryo transfer technique used may influence implantation rates. Despite improvements in ART, the reproductive success rates – seen as an ongoing pregnancy or a healthy live birth – are still low; clinical pregnancy rates remains around 35 percent per transfer and MPR is 17 percent per transfer (10) owing to the challenge of choosing the embryo with the highest implantation potential.

Evaluation of the embryo cohort depends on the skill of the embryologists, who ultimately, decide which embryo will be transferred. Embryo evaluation at determined time-points is a nonspecific and highly subjective selection method. Embryo selection based on morphological assessment at D5 may not always identify the best embryo for transfer, therefore reducing implantation and pregnancy rates.

The new paradigm in ART is to offer a personalized IVF treatment for patients aimed at increasing the chance of a live birth. Specifically, treatment individualization is also applicable in embryo-selection techniques. Various techniques have been developed to identify and select objectively the best embryo in the cohort for transfer and to obtain the highest probability of success. Technologies and strategies such as the development of new algorithms for embryo selection, genetic screening, and the determination of embryo energy potential are some examples.

8.5 Preimplantation Genetic Test for Aneuploidies (PGT-A)

Ploidy of the embryo plays a very important role in the development of embryos, as well as in their implantation potential. The incidence of aneuploidy in human gametes increase with age, especially in women. Oocyte aneuploidy rates exceed 50 percent for most women over 40 years. Consequently, over half of embryos can carry chromosomal abnormalities.

Preimplantation genetic tests are effective screening tools to evaluate the embryo's chromosome complement. Numerical (PGT-A) and structural (PGT-SR) chromosomal abnormalities are related to poor blastocyst quality, implantation failure, miscarriage, and poor clinical pregnancy outcomes (5).

Genetic analysis can be performed in different cell types. Polar body biopsy allows a detailed testing of the maternal genome in a less invasive form for the embryo, as the embryo itself is not affected by removing half of the oocyte's genetic material. However, this technique does not permit the analysis of the paternal genetic contribution and the existence of genetic errors which occurred in early embryo development (12).

Cleavage or blastocyst-stage embryo biopsy became more popular for their accuracy in predicting aneuploidies in the embryo (91 and 94 percent, respectively), thus both progenitor's meiotic errors will be detected (13). The genetic screening in blastomere at D3 shows an improvement of clinical outcomes and has the benefit that the embryo can be transferred in blastocyst stage in a fresh cycle. Nonetheless, the cleavage-stage biopsy may alter embryo development and reduce its implantation potential of 39 percent, compared to nonbiopsied embryos (12, 13).

While cleavage-stage biopsy is harmful for the embryo (removing one-sixth or one-eighth of the embryo), blastocyst-stage biopsy seems to be safe. Although it is a highly invasive technique, the capability of analyzing embryo ploidy is higher. The number of cells retrieved in trophectoderm biopsy is higher, so more DNA is available for analysis compared to cleavage-stage biopsy in which only one blastomere can be used. This improves the accuracy of genetic testing.

Various studies have evaluated the clinical impact of blastocyst biopsy, concluding that IVF outcomes were improved without compromising implantation rate, ongoing pregnancy, and delivery rates when compared with unbiopsied embryos (12). Unlike cleavage-stage biopsy, trophectoderm biopsy requires a high-quality vitrification protocol owing to the time required for genetic analysis, giving that the embryo transfer has to be performed on D5 or D6 (13).

The advancement of technology has allowed the creation of more accurate genetic tests that are capable of analyzing the entire chromosomal complement of cells. Traditionally, fluorescent in situ hybridization (FISH) was widely used for chromosome screening but has the limitation that only a small number of chromosomes can be analyzed simultaneously. PGT analysis with FISH does not confer any advantage for infertile couples with a poor chance of conceiving (it had no effect on live birth rates) (12, 14).

Comprehensive chromosome screening (CCS) is a new genetic testing method which analyzes whole chromosome complements. This technique can be applied at different stages of embryonic development and it can be performed with the use of different genetic platforms, like comparative genomic hybridization (CGH), single-nucleotide polymorphism (SNP) and next-generation sequencing (NGS) (12, 14).

PGT-A is employed in IVF cycles in different scenarios where the risk of embryo aneuploidy is high, e.g., advanced maternal age, parental balanced-chromosomal aberrations, recurrent pregnancy loss, severe male factor infertility or repeated implantation failure. The classical embryo selection based on morphology cannot be used as an alternative to genetic screening to minimize the risk of transferring chromosomally abnormal embryos (5).

Traditionally, the widespread strategy has been MET with the aim to bypass the reduced implantation potential of possibly aneuploid embryos and achieving at least one single live birth; however, this practice is associated with high MPR. Recently, PGT-A at blastocyst stage has been proposed as a tool to improve embryo selection in SET cycles, coupled with the morphologic assessment.

PGT-A is an objective embryo-selection method that has been used to avoid the transfer of abnormal, nonviable embryos; the transmission of chromosomal errors to the offspring; and to improve clinical outcomes. Embryo selection based on euploidy can significantly improve implantation rates in women of advanced maternal age, with a significant increase in live birth rates (LBR) per embryo transfer for SET/PGT-A cycles (15).

The most recent meta-analyses and reviews agree that PGT-A using CCS at blastocyst stage improves embryo selection and increases implantation rates in IVF cycles in patients with good prognosis (14, 16). Nevertheless, there is a lack of RCTs evaluating the clinical outcomes of euploid SET in women with poor reproductive prognosis. This is remarkable, especially as this patient population is very common in IVF clinics. Further research is needed to find the best SET strategy for this subgroup of patients.

Efficiency of genetic aneuploidy screening is reduced by embryo mosaicism, as different cell lines – euploid and aneuploid – may be present in the embryo. The prevalence of embryo mosaicism is relatively high but the implantation potential is reduced; besides, it is important to exclude mosaic embryos in PGT-A analyses (13). The understanding of this limiting factor is critical in order to choose the best embryo stage to perform the biopsy, bearing in mind that there is more likelihood to detect mosaicism in blastocysts.

Although clinical results are improved when PGT-A is performed compared to solely morphology-based embryo selection, the embryo biopsy is a highly invasive procedure which can affect embryo development and may not be available at every laboratory. In addition, genetic analysis generates ethical and moral considerations and it is not permissible in some countries. Furthermore, the cost-effectiveness of PGT-A should be taken into consideration owing to the increase in the cost of IVF treatments when it is applied. Nonetheless, PGT-A has the power to maximize both, the clinical and economic benefits of ART cycles, resulting in a singleton baby in a shorter period of time (16).

In the near future, genetic analysis may be possible in a noninvasive manner using the cell-free DNA (cfDNA), released by embryos into the culture medium (so-called spent medium). This new clinical approach has been studied by different groups to evaluate the sensitivity and specificity of cfDNA to determine embryo aneuploidy. One of the latest prospective pilot studies found high sensitivity and specificity values (94.5 percent and 71.7 percent, respectively) when the embryonic cfDNA was analyzed at D6/7 (with high ploidy concordance with TE biopsy results) (17). In addition, cfDNA analysis would determine the impact of embryo mosaicism, as all the genetic content is released by the embryo rather than the analysis being carried out on a small set of cells.

8.6 Time-Lapse Monitoring Systems

One of the new strategies to improve embryo selection, and thereby increase the success rate after embryo transfer, is the use of time-lapse (TL) technology. The image-acquisition system may be integrated in embryo incubators like EmbryoScope (Vitrolife), Geri (Genea Biomedex) (both with their improved Plus versions) or Miri TL (Esco Medical) or may be inserted in a conventional incubator such as the Eeva Test (Merk Serono) or Primo Vision (Vitrolife) (Figure 8.2).

Time-lapse monitoring systems allow the continuous recording of embryo development without adverse effects on the embryos. The acquisition of multiple images in short time intervals (5–15 minutes) enables the observation of developmental events and the evaluation of the morphologic parameters, starting from the early stages of embryo development. This technology has expanded worldwide owing to the advantages that TL systems have over traditional incubators.

	Tokai-hit®	PrimoVision®	Eeva®	Geri®	Miri®	ES +®
System	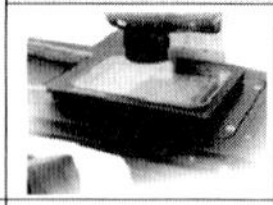	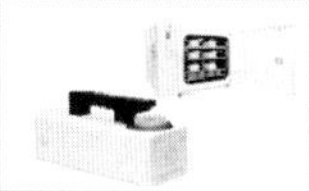	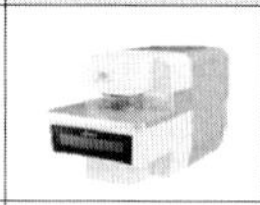	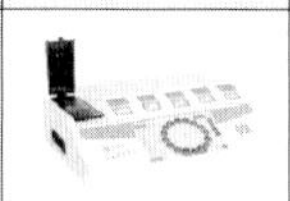	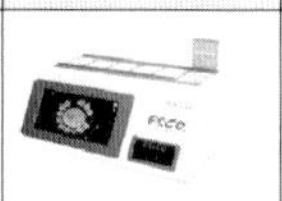	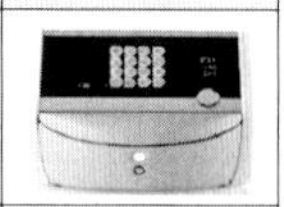
Dishes	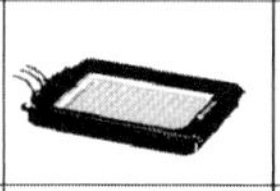	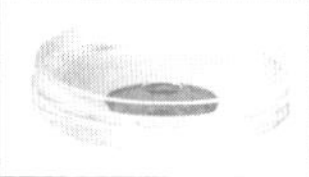	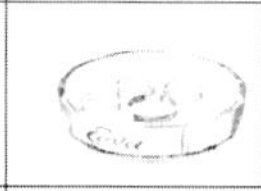	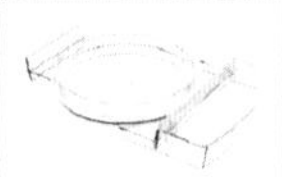	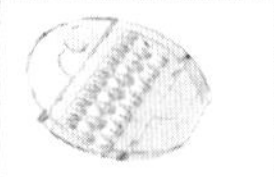	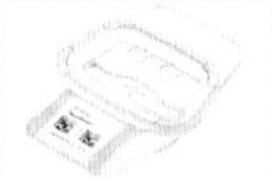
Optics	Bright field	Bright field	Dark field	Bright/Dark field	Bright field	Bright field
Embryos	6/12/24/48/96 wells	16 embryo/dish	12 embryo/dish	16 embryo/dish	14 embryo/dish	16 embryo/dish
Dishes	1 multi-well	1 d/camera	1 d/camera	6 d/system	6 d/system	15 d/system

Figure 8.2 Types of time-lapse systems and their main characteristics: an incubator built over a microscope (Tokai-hit), microscopes built inside incubators (PrimoVision and Eeva), and systems consisting of a microscope and an incubator (Geri, Miri, and EmbryoScope Plus, ES+).

Briefly, this technology facilitates the evaluation of embryos from a dynamic point of view, providing kinetic information on embryo development. The culture conditions are highly controlled, as it is not necessary to remove embryos from the incubator for their evaluation – a process which may impair embryo development. Finally, objective information is obtained, quantitatively as well as qualitatively.

In addition, as classical morphology embryo evaluation is made at only few time points, certain abnormal events might be missed, e.g., direct cleavage (DC: direct 1–3 cells <5 hours), reverse cleavage (RC: 3–2 cell embryo), irregular cells divisions and multinucleation (presence of two or more nucleus in interphase). These events have been related to poor embryo quality and reduced implantation potential (18, 19). The information collected by TL microscopy provides several biomarkers currently under investigation, which can act as an embryo selection or deselection tool in a noninvasive form (18).

The timescale of embryonic development has been used for kinetic parameters which, in conjunction with embryo morphology evaluation (called morphokinetic parameters), allows the creation of algorithms to select the best embryo. With TL technology, the morphokinetic parameters are annotated in a software package to establish an embryo-grading system based on the implantation potential (Figure 8.3). Thus, embryos are sorted in a hierarchical ranking according to the best quality characteristics and reproductive prognosis, allowing more precise decisions on which embryo will be transferred in a SET cycle.

The earliest studies performed with EmbryoScope (ESD) incubators identified important morphokinetic parameters and led to the development of different embryo-selection algorithms. The duration of the first cytokinesis and second cell cycle, the time between second and third cell cycle, the time of division to five cells, and the time intervals between 2–8 cell and 5–8 cell stages are some examples of new kinetic markers. Moreover, these parameters were correlated with embryo development to blastocyst stage and implantation potential, which are clinical outcomes of IVF cycles (12, 18, 20).

Other studies focused on the relationship between cell cycle characteristics and embryo ploidy. Although morphological assessment has limited success at identifying euploid

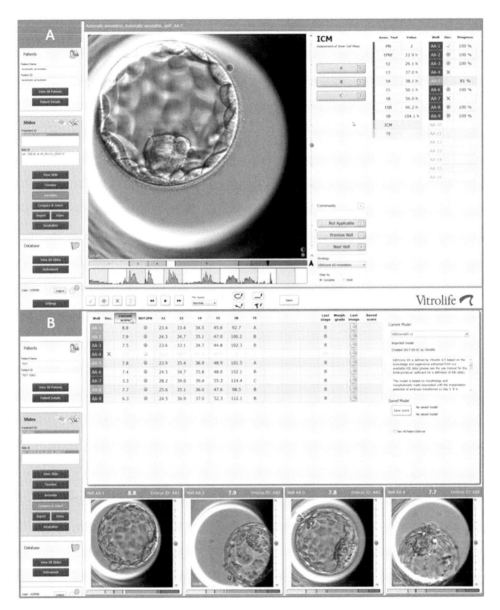

Figure 8.3 EmbryoScope software (EmbryoViewer, Copenhagen, Vitrolife). (A) Annotations of morphokinetic and morphological variables performed semiautomatically during the embryo development based on the algorithm KID score d5 v.2. (B) Classification of an embryo cohort based on the algorithm KID Score d5 v.2, according to the implantation potential. The higher the score, the better.

embryos, and PGT is an invasive technique which may harm embryos, several groups proposed TL technology as a predictive and noninvasive tool of embryo aneuploidy and implantation potential.

The initial hypothesis – that euploid embryos have better kinetic profiles in their development compared to aneuploid embryos – was confirmed in some studies. Differences in the morphokinetic behavior during early stages of development were found between normal and abnormal embryos. Based on these results, algorithms were developed with the aim of selecting embryos with a higher probability of chromosomal normality (12, 19, 20).

Nevertheless, other groups failed to correlate the morphokinetic parameters with embryo ploidy status, and were not able to segregate euploid embryos from aneuploid embryos. These groups advocated genetic screening as the only reliable technique to determine the chromosomal status of embryos, which cannot be replaced with an embryo-selection algorithm based on morphokinetics (12, 19, 20). However, a genetic test – ideally noninvasive – would complement the embryo selection by morphokinetic parameters, and by combining both parameters increase the confidence of the embryologist when deciding which is the best embryo to transfer in SET cycles in cases where more than one euploid blastocyst is available.

Despite the advantages offered by embryo culture in TL incubators and the creation of different embryo-selection algorithms, none is universally accepted. There are few RCTs that validate their clinical use. Owing to the existence of confounding factors affecting embryo development (such as heterogeneous populations, different culture conditions, type of IVF treatment), widespread clinical implementation is complex. The creation of in-house selection algorithms for each clinic, considering its own particularities, should increase the predictive capacity of TL as an embryo-selection tool.

Machine learning (ML) and artificial intelligence (AI) may improve the assessment of embryo development in the future. AI is the development of computer systems capable of performing human intelligence's own tasks. With the ML and deep learning, a computer can learn from input data to develop its own mechanism of processing unstructured or unlabeled new data and creating patterns for use in decision-making. The large amount of data generated by TL systems permits the application of AI (19) for impartial and automated evaluation of embryos. This revolutionary approach reduces human variability in embryo assessment and improves objective embryo selection.

Artificial intelligence systems provide accurate quality assessments in different clinical conditions. Specifically, in IVF treatments it is important to correlate the embryo quality with good clinical outcomes to improve success rates. In this sense, one of these new approaches can predict blastocyst quality without human intervention, calculated by an area under the curve (AUC) >98. Furthermore, the system shows the chance of pregnancy (based on individual embryos) depending on automated embryo quality evaluation and the mother's age (21).

Artificial intelligence could also be used to improve the efficacy of embryo assessment performed by standard morphology or the existing algorithms based on morphokinetic parameters. Additionally, analysis of morphokinetics and/or images by AI could be a potential tool to select which embryo is to be transferred, vitrified, or discarded.

8.7 Mitoscore

The objective selection of the embryo with the highest implantation potential, especially in SET cycles when several euploid blastocysts are available, is today's goal in IVF. However, a proportion of the morphologically and chromosomally normal embryos, which are transferred, fail to implant. One of the possible causes of this fact is an energy deficit and impaired functionality of the mitochondria, which affect embryonic developmental ability.

Mitochondria are small organelles involved in multiple essential processes in the eukaryotic cell, but the generation of cell energy in the form of adenosine triphosphate (ATP) by oxidative phosphorylation is their main function. Its size and number vary between different cell types and depends on the energetic needs of each cell (22).

One of the differential characteristics of mitochondria is that they are the only organelles that have their own genome. The mitochondrial DNA (mtDNA) is a circular, double-strand genome which codifies several genes related to cellular metabolism, oxidative phosphorylation, and some of the components of transcriptional and translational cell machinery like 22 tRNAs and 2 rRNAs. The mtDNA is replicated independently of nuclear genome and its value is indicative for the mitochondria number in the cell (23).

The oocyte is the cell in woman's body with the largest number of both mitochondria and mtDNA. Mitochondrial replication begins during fetal development and continues until the oocyte is arrested in metaphase II stage, when the germ cell contains approximately 100,000 mitochondria and more than 500,000 mtDNA copies. Thus, the mtDNA units that the early embryo possesses are the initial amount stored in the unfertilized oocyte, since mitochondrial inheritance is exclusively maternal (bottleneck mechanism) (24). As a result, during embryo divisions the total mtDNA is split among cells, diluting the initial mtDNA concentration (25).

No additional mtDNA expansion occurs from fertilization until D5. From the blastocyst stage onward, energy production is up-regulated in order to support cell differentiation into trophectoderm and inner cell mass and the later postimplantation development of the embryo (22, 23).

The mtDNA content in oocytes and embryos has been studied with the purpose of finding a biomarker for embryo selection correlated with the embryo's potential to lead to pregnancies and live births. Several studies have attempted to find a relationship between mtDNA levels with embryo viability, maternal age, embryo chromosomal status, and implantation potential.

There is controversial evidence that there is a connection between maternal age and the amount of mtDNA stored in oocytes (24). Lower levels of mtDNA were found in oocytes with incomplete cytoplasmic maturation, in degenerated oocytes, and in those from infertile women with diminished ovarian reserve.

Measuring the mtDNA levels could be a tool to evaluate embryo quality. As the concentration of mtDNA is diluted among cells with each embryonic division, lower levels would be associated with better embryo quality and an improvement of clinical outcomes (24) (Figure 8.4). The mtDNA copy number was quantified by real-time polymerase chain reaction (RT-PCR), taking into account the amount of nuclear DNA (nDNA) of the cells to normalize the mtDNA content. Its measurement can be made from the cells collected in the embryo biopsy. The ratio of mtDNA/nDNA is called the mitochondrial score (Ms) or Mitoscore (25). The Ms value represents the relative mtDNA copy number per cell, and can be used as an indicator of energy distress and embryo viability.

The power of Ms to evaluate embryo viability was considered in a retrospective study from the clinical outcome (measured as implantation rate) of euploid SET (25). A high mtDNA value was related to a poor implantation potential: the mtDNA content for cleavage embryos that successfully implanted was statistically lower than those that did not. In addition, the Ms value at blastocyst stage showed the same result.

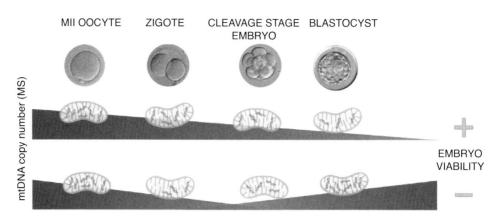

Figure 8.4 Relationship between embryo viability and mitochondrial DNA (mtDNA). The concentration of mtDNA is diluted among cells with each embryonic division, and this would be associated with better embryo quality. Adapted from Cecchino and García-Velasco (24). A black and white version of this figure will appear in some formats. For the colour version, please refer to the plate section.

Based on these data, the mitochondrial score was used to predict the implantation potential of euploid embryos, taking into account their mtDNA copy number. In addition, the Ms value was related to recurrent miscarriage and advanced maternal age, finding a trend toward an increase of Ms score in poorer quality embryos. However, only euploid embryos were analyzed, which is an important limitation to the study (25).

Another study also found a clear association between mtDNA levels and embryo implantation potential (23). Higher blastocyst implantation rates were linked to lower mtDNA amounts; a threshold of the relative Ms was detected, after which embryos never implanted (with a 100 percent negative predictive value for embryo implantation potential).

On the other hand, significant differences in mtDNA content were found in embryos from older women, demonstrating the aging effect in oocyte and embryo quality, and between euploid and aneuploid embryos, when obtained from women of the same age. It is not known if the chromosomal abnormalities cause the increased mtDNA number in the embryos or whether these two factor are independent and the real cause is still undefined (23).

Both results (23, 25) are in accordance to "the quiet embryo hypothesis," which is based on the idea that stress could impair embryo development owing to an overactivated metabolism, whereas most viable embryos have a lower metabolism. Those embryos with energy deficiencies may suffer metabolic distress resulting in an increase of both mitochondrial activation and mtDNA replication in order to compensate the energy demanded (24). This energetic stress may be related to defective oocyte maturation, impaired respiratory capacities, mtDNA mutations, aging, or oxidative stress, among other factors.

A recent study evaluated whether the Ms may correlate with the kinetic parameters of embryonic development and ploidy status in cleavage-stage embryos (22). The mtDNA content was measured in blastomeres to stratify in two groups (low and high Ms) and to compare between them. The number of euploid embryos was equal in both groups (in contrast to previous results) and the Ms value was not different between them with the same blastomere number.

Embryo monitoring with time-lapse technology allows the evaluation of the embryo's kinetic parameters. The embryos in the low Mitoscore group presented a significantly higher cell number on D3 and they reached the eight-cell stage faster. Moreover, the absence of cavitation when blastocyst formation occurred (within 118 hours of embryo development) was correlated with higher Ms values and a lower chance of being chromosomally normal (22).

The mitochondrial DNA copy number is an index of embryonic energetic stress that could indicate a decreased amount of metabolic fuel which finally may affect the embryo's implantation capacity. The Ms value has been correlated with good-quality embryos in terms of a higher chance of being euploid and an increased implantation potential when the Ms value is low. However, most studies published to date are retrospective, with small and heterogeneous populations among them, and, at the moment, there is no standardized technique to measure mtDNA levels, which poses an important bias in this approach.

This novel technique to evaluate the embryonic potential seems a promising approach to select the embryo with the best characteristics to transfer and the highest chance to achieve a viable pregnancy; however, more research is required to understand better the true clinical utility of Ms as a biomarker of embryo viability.

8.8 Summary

To date, despite all the improvements achieved in ART, many couples are unable to achieve pregnancy and birth of a healthy child. The ultimate goal of IVF treatment is to select the single best embryo out of the cohort to transfer, avoiding multiple embryo transfer and, therefore, reducing multiple gestations.

The improvement of clinical success goes hand-in-hand with novel embryo-selection methods that have been developed with the aim to choose the embryo in an objective way. All the above techniques have demonstrated their value to select with more confidence the embryo with the best characteristics and higher potential to achieve a live birth.

Genetic preimplantation testing allows differentiation between chromosomally abnormal and normal embryos; the embryo-selection algorithms classify embryos from their morphokinetic parameters based on the implantation potential; and the Ms value is a reflection of embryo mitochondrial content, which correlates with their implantation potential.

Traditional morphological embryo selection should be coupled with these tools for the purpose of choosing the preeminent single embryo that has the highest chances of implanting. These techniques show promise but it is still necessary for them to be proven as effective and harmless before their widespread use in clinical practice.

References

1. Glujovsky D, Farquhar C, Am QR, et al. Cleavage stage versus blastocyst stage embryo transfer in assisted reproductive technology: summary of findings for the main comparison. Cochrane Database Syst Rev 2016;30:CD002118.

2. Maheshwari A, Hamilton M, Bhattacharya S. Should we be promoting embryo transfer at blastocyst stage? Reprod Biomed Online 2016;32:142–146.

3. Practice Committees of the American Society for Reproductive Medicine and the Society. Blastocyst culture and transfer in

clinically assisted reproduction: a committee opinion. Fertil Steril 2018;110:1246–1252.

4. Alpha Scientists in Reproductive Medicine and ESHRE Special Interest Group of Embryology. The Istanbul consensus workshop on embryo assessment: proceedings of an expert meeting. Hum Reprod 2011;26:1270–1283.

5. Capalbo A, Rienzi L, Cimadomo D, et al. Correlation between standard blastocyst morphology, euploidy and implantation: an observational study in two centers involving 956 screened blastocysts. Hum Reprod 2014;29:1173–1181.

6. Cutting R. Single embryo transfer for all. Best Pract Res Clin Obstet Gynaecol 2018;53:30–37.

7. Pandian Z, Marjoribanks J, Ozturk O, et al. Number of embryos for transfer following in vitro fertilisation or intra-cytoplasmic sperm injection: summary of a Cochrane review. Fertil Steril 2014;102:345–347.

8. Wilkinson D, Schaefer GO, Tremellen K, et al. Double trouble: should double embryo transfer be banned? Theor Med Bioeth 2015;36:121–139.

9. Harbottle S, Hughes C, Cutting R, et al. Elective single embryo transfer: an update to UK Best Practice Guidelines. Hum Fertil 2015;18:165–183.

10. De Geyter C, Calhaz-Jorge C, Kupka MS, et al. ART in Europe, 2014: results generated from European registries by ESHRE. Hum Reprod 2018;33:1586–1601.

11. Practice Committee of the American Society for Reproductive Medicine and Practice Committee of the Society for Assisted Reproductive Technology. Criteria for number of embryos to transfer: a committee opinion. Fertil Steril 2013;99:44–46.

12. Sigalos G, Triantafyllidou O, Vlahos NF. Novel embryo selection techniques to increase embryo implantation in IVF attempts. Arch Gynecol Obstet 2016;294:1117–1124.

13. Scott KL, Hong KH, Scott RT Jr. Selecting the optimal time to perform biopsy for preimplantation genetic testing. Fertil Steril 2013;100:608–614.

14. Dahdouh EM, Sc M, Balayla J, et al. Comprehensive chromosome screening improves embryo selection: a meta-analysis. Fertil Steril 2015;104:1503–1512.

15. Ubaldi FM, Capalbo A, Colamaria S, et al. Reduction of multiple pregnancies in the advanced maternal age population after implementation of an elective single embryo transfer policy coupled with enhanced embryo selection: pre- and post-intervention study. Hum Reprod 2015;30:2097–2106.

16. Lee E, Illingworth P, Wilton L, et al. The clinical effectiveness of preimplantation genetic diagnosis for aneuploidy in all 24 chromosomes (PGD-A): systematic review. Hum Reprod 2015;30:473–483.

17. Rubio C, Rienzi L, Navarro-Sánchez L, et al. Embryonic cell-free DNA versus trophectoderm biopsy for aneuploidy testing: concordance rate and clinical implications. Fertil Steril 2019;112:510–519.

18. Castelló D, Motato Y, Basile N, et al. How much have we learned from time-lapse in clinical IVF? Mol Hum Reprod 2016;22:719–727.

19. Del Gallego R, Remohí J, Meseguer M. Time-lapse imaging: the state of the art. Biol Reprod 2019;101:1146–1154.

20. Kirkegaard K, Ahlström A, Ingerslev HJ, et al. Choosing the best embryo by time lapse versus standard morphology. Fertil Steril 2015;103:323–332.

21. Khosravi P, Kazemi E, Zhan Q, et al. Deep learning enables robust assessment and selection of human blastocysts after in vitro fertilization. npj Digit Med 2019;2:21. doi:10.1038/s41746-019-0096-y.

22. Bayram A, De Munck N, Elkhatib I, et al. Cleavage stage mitochondrial DNA is correlated with preimplantation human embryo development and ploidy status. J Assist Reprod Genet 2019;36:1847–1854.

23. Fragouli E, Spath K, Alfarawati S, et al. Altered Levels of Mitochondrial DNA Are

Associated with Female Age, Aneuploidy, and Provide an Independent Measure of Embryonic Implantation Potential. PLoS Genet 2015;11:E1005241.

24. Cecchino GN, García-Velasco JA. Mitochondrial DNA copy number as a predictor of embryo viability. Fertil Steril 2019;111:205–211.

25. Diez-Juan A, Rubio C, Marin C, et al. DNA content as a viability score in human euploid embryos: less is better. Fertil Steril 2015;104:534–541.

Preparation for Optimal Endometrial Receptivity in Cryo Cycles

Carol Coughlan, Barbara Lawrenz, and Human M. Fatemi

9.1 Background

Despite the various advances and increasing success rates of assisted conception treatment in recent years, implantation continues to be a rate limiting step (1). The first successful IVF treatment performed by the pioneers Patrick Steptoe and Robert Edwards which led to the birth of Louise Joy Brown in 1978, was achieved in a fresh embryo transfer cycle. The subsequent implementation of cryopreservation techniques in the IVF laboratory facilitated the cryopreservation and storage of supernumerary embryos which were not chosen for a fresh transfer. Laboratory techniques have improved significantly over the years and due to the improved survival rates of cryopreserved oocytes, cleavage, and blastocyst-stage embryos, cryopreservation of gametes and embryos has become part of everyday routine clinical practice (2).

Many factors have contributed to the increase in embryo freezing in ART practice worldwide (3). There is no doubt as to the benefit to couples of cryopreservation of surplus oocytes or embryos. IVF treatment poses not only a significant emotional and physical burden but also takes a financial toll on the affected couple and limited financial resources may result in couples having to abandon treatment prematurely. Cryopreservation of surplus oocytes or embryos offers the couple the opportunity to increase their cumulative chance of pregnancy without necessitating further ovarian stimulation cycles.

Over the past four decades, advances in cancer therapies particularly chemotherapeutics, have led to dramatic improvements in patient survival. Given that more patients are surviving their cancer, care is increasingly expanding to include improving long-term health and quality of life. One of the most important quality of life issues in reproductive-age cancer survivors is the ability to have biological children. Vitrification of oocytes and embryos and, more recently, ovarian tissue cryopreservation allow patients the opportunity to preserve their fertility in advance of commencing cytotoxic treatments (4).

In recent years, we have seen a steady increase in the number of patients opting to freeze oocytes or embryos due to social reasons (5). In addition, to facilitate preimplantation genetic testing for aneuploidy (PGT-A) at blastocyst stage, cycle segmentation with vitrification of the embryo and subsequent frozen embryo transfer is required due to the necessary turn-around time of genetic testing results and the limited window of implantation (6). The current testing method of day 5 multiple cell trophectoderm biopsy, next-generation sequencing (NGS) and 24 chromosome screening has resulted in significantly improved implantation rates as compared to the initial day 3 single blastomere biopsy and the initial genetic testing method FISH (fluorescence in situ hybridization (FISH). With the increasing practice of embryo cryopreservation worldwide arises the question what is the optimal cycle regimen for frozen embryo transfer cycles? The aim of this review is to summarize and critically appraise the existing data comparing different approaches to endometrial preparation for frozen embryo transfer (FET).

9.2 Endometrial Receptivity

For implantation to occur, a blastocyst must attach to and invade the endometrium under the influence of both estrogen and progesterone (Figure 9.1). Endometrial receptivity is driven by the secretory transformation of the endometrium under the influence of progesterone following estrogen exposure. In humans, the exact duration of the window of implantation is difficult to define. In an idealized 28-day cycle, it is assumed to take place between day 19 and day 21 of the menstrual cycle, with a described duration of 48 hours up to 4 days (7–11). The daily histological changes occurring under the influence of progesterone, have been described as long ago as 1950 by Noyes et al. (12).

In fresh, as well as in frozen embryo transfers a receptive endometrium, a good-quality, euploid embryo and synchrony between the endometrium and embryo development stage are crucial to achieve a pregnancy. The most common treatment protocols for frozen embryo transfers include natural cycles with or without HCG trigger or endometrial preparation with hormonal treatment (artificial cycles), with or without gonadotrophin – releasing hormone agonist suppression.

There is ongoing controversy regarding the optimal means to prepare the endometrium for frozen embryo transfer (FET) cycles. Numerous studies have compared the implantation and pregnancy rates in fresh embryo transfer cycles (fresh ET) to FET (frozen embryo transfer cycles) and between the different approaches taken to prepare the endometrium for FET. Accuracy in the timing of embryo transfer following progesterone exposure is critical to the success of frozen embryo transfers. If the timing of embryo transfer in FET cycles

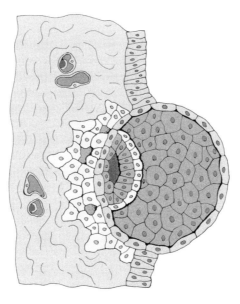

Figure 9.1 Diagrammatic representation of embryo implantation. A black and white version of this figure will appear in some formats. For the colour version, please refer to the plate section.

included in these scientific studies is inaccurate, then the conclusions drawn from these studies will also be inaccurate.

9.2.1 Timing of FET in a Natural Cycle

In contrast to a HRT cycle where follicle growth and spontaneous ovulation result in cycle cancellation, in a natural cycle estrogen and progesterone production from a dominant follicle and subsequently from the corpus luteum are crucial for endometrial preparation. In a natural cycle, estradiol synthesis increases progressively from the dominant follicle and initiates the LH surge. Prior to the LH surge, a small increase in progesterone level is seen, which reflects the increasing LH pulse amplitude and frequency leading up to the surge. An LH surge of 24–36 hours is sufficient to initiate the resumption of oocyte meiosis, luteinization of granulosa cells, ovulation, and the initial phase of corpora lutea development. Progesterone and 17α-hydroxyprogesterone (17α-OHP) plasma concentrations increase rapidly after the LH surge indicating the beginning of granulosa and theca cell luteinization (13). The corpus luteum produces up to 40 mg of progesterone per day in addition to a significant quantity of androgens and estradiol (14).

Following the pathophysiology of natural conception, the embryo is deemed to arrive in the uterine cavity approximately five days after fertilization of the oocyte by the sperm in the fallopian tube while the aforementioned hormonal changes prepare the receptive endometrium for implantation. The process of implantation, which involves embryo apposition, attachment to the maternal endometrial epithelium and invasion into the endometrial stroma can only occur when the endometrium is receptive (Figure 9.1) (15). This phase is commonly referred to as the "window of implantation" (WOI) (15–17).

FET can be planned in a pure natural cycle (NC) in patients with regular spontaneous ovulatory cycles or in a modified natural cycle (mNC), using hCG (Human Chorionic Gonadotropin) for ovulation induction. In a natural cycle, follicle growth and spontaneous ovulation are crucial for endometrial preparation. The key to success of embryo transfer in a natural cycle is the accurate detection of the LH surge and subsequent ovulation in order to determine the timing of the embryo transfer accurately. As described above, the LH surge in a natural cycle is initiated through increasing estradiol levels, produced by the growing dominant follicle. When the LH concentration rises by 180 percent above the most recent serum values and continues to rise thereafter, the LH surge is considered to have begun (18). As a consequence of rising LH levels, luteinization of granulosa cells, and synthesis of progesterone is stimulated and a drop in estradiol levels follows the initiation of the LH surge. When LH surge, ovulation, and the rise of progesterone levels are confirmed by blood tests, subsequently the embryo transfer has to be planned according to the embryo development stage at the time of embryo freezing/vitrification. Figure 9.2 depicts the hormonal constellation of estradiol (E2), progesterone (P4) and LH to identify the LH surge and the day of ovulation.

Detection of the LH surge and the estradiol decrease in blood requires frequent patient visits to the clinic, therefore the use of urinary LH kits to detect ovulation may seem to be a more patient-friendly and convenient approach in a natural cycle. However, the use of urinary LH kits have several disadvantages which may result in incorrect identification of the LH surge. LH levels in the urine follow the serum peak by nearly 24 hours because of the required time for urinary LH clearance (19). In addition, urinary LH kits may demonstrate LH surges in the absence of ovulation (20) and finally a high percentage of normally cycling

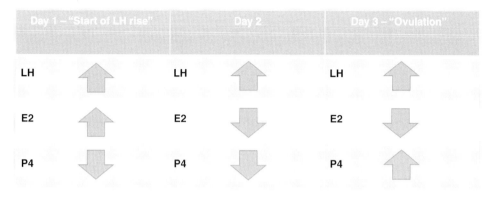

Day 1 – "Start of LH rise"		Day 2		Day 3 – "Ovulation"	
LH	⬆	LH	⬆	LH	⬆
E2	⬆	E2	⬇	E2	⬇
P4	⬇	P4	⬇	P4	⬆

Figure 9.2 Hormonal constellation to identify the LH surge and the day of ovulation.

women may demonstrate premature LH surges which do not trigger ovulation and therefore if a clinician depends solely on urinary LH kits to identify the LH surge it is very likely that the timing of embryo transfer will be inaccurate and result in an unsuccessful cycle (20, 21). It is worth bearing in mind that the conclusions of studies using LH urinary kits to determine timing of the LH surge have to be evaluated critically and may not be scientifically accurate.

9.2.2 Timing of FET in Hormonal Replacement Cycle

The advantages of a HRT-FET cycle are obvious: first, disturbances due to cycle variation can be avoided, second, the number of patient visits to the clinic for ultrasound scans and hormonal monitoring can be reduced and third, this approach facilitates flexibility with scheduling of the embryo transfer procedure which is an advantage for both the clinic and patient.

In a hormonal replacement therapy (HRT) cycle for FET, the hormonal changes of a natural cycle are simulated by commencing estradiol administration on the second or third day of the cycle and continuing throughout the cycle to promote endometrial development. When a sufficient endometrial thickness is confirmed by ultrasound examination, progesterone is introduced to induce secretory transformation of the endometrium. The critical step in a HRT-FET cycle is to adjust the duration of progesterone exposure to the developmental stage of the embryo following estradiol administration to prepare the endometrium. Theoretically, progesterone can be administered orally, rectally, subcutaneously, vaginally, and via the intramuscular route with the two latter modes of administration being the most commonly applied in clinical practice (22). The serum progesterone's rise and it´s subsequent effect on the endometrium vary depending on the route of progesterone administration.

Progesterone is rapidly absorbed after intramuscular (IM) injection and higher doses will result in earlier and higher peak serum levels: following injection of 25 mg, 50 mg, and 100 mg of progesterone, peak concentrations were 16.9 ng/mL, 36.5 ng/mL, and 83.8 ng/mL, respectively, and these peak levels were attained 5 hours after injection of the 25 mg and 50 mg dosage and 3.5 hours following the injection of the 100 mg dose. Thirteen hours after the injection, progesterone plasma levels decreased to 10.9 ng/mL (25 mg), 19.8 ng/mL (50 mg), and 40.7 ng/mL (100 mg), respectively (23).

In contrast to the rapidly increasing serum progesterone levels following IM injection, serum progesterone concentrations reach maximal levels two to four hours after vaginal application of a 400 mg suppository with a maximum peak of 35 ng/mL (24). It is well recognized that vaginal absorption of progesterone is enhanced following previous estrogenization (25).

Despite low serum progesterone levels, adequate secretory endometrial transformation is achieved by vaginally administered progesterone. This suggests a direct local effect on the endometrium before entering the systemic circulation, the so-called first uterine pass effect.

HRT-FET can be performed with or without co-treatment with a GnRH (Gonadotropin-Releasing-Hormone) analog. Incorporating a GnRH analog into the treatment protocol reduces the risk of cycle cancellation due to spontaneous ovulation which may occur despite the administration of exogenous hormones. The advantages of employing this approach include a reduction in the number of patient visits to the clinic for ultrasound and hormonal monitoring, cycle cancellations due to cycle variation can be avoided, and this approach facilitates embryo transfer planning.

9.2.3   Is the "True NC-FET" in the Literature Really "True"?

Data on the efficacy of a "true" NC-FET cycle compared to a HRT-FET are limited. Previous studies have focused for the most part on modified natural cycles using human chorionic gonadotrophin to induce ovulation of the dominant follicle which has been shown to be inferior to a spontaneous natural cycle for planning of frozen-thawed embryo transfer (26). Administration of hCG in the late follicular phase induces changes in the endometrium, which would have occurred several days later in a natural cycle (26). In addition, human chorionic gonadotrophin (hCG) and LH act on the endometrium through the same receptor and it has been suggested that their simultaneous presence may have an adverse effect on pregnancy rates (26, 27). Cochrane meta-analyzes, comparing different FET approaches, were published in 2008 and 2017 both concluding that there is insufficient evidence to support the use of one cycle regimen in preference to another in preparation for FET in subfertile women with regular ovulatory cycles (28, 29). The overall quality of the evidence was very poor in both meta-analyses. The main limitation was poor reporting of study methods. In addition, the studies referenced as studies of the natural cycle in the 2017 analysis were essentially abstracts and never published as full papers (30, 31). It also has to be noted that the study by Karimzadeh et al., did not meet the criteria for a "true" NC-FET as hCG was used for ovulation induction which has been clearly shown to be significantly less effective as compared to a true natural cycle (31).

A recent study comparing artificial and natural cycles concluded that the optimal means of endometrial preparation for frozen-thawed cycle remains unclear and both options may be offered to women with regular ovulatory cycles in line with the previous Cochrane meta-analyses (32). However this study identified ovulation based on ultrasound findings alone which means that a premature LH or progesterone rise would be missed leading to inaccurate timing of ovulation. In addition, the natural cycle was modified by the use of hCG to induce ovulation which has been shown to be inferior to a spontaneous natural cycle (26). A further recent systematic review and meta-analysis of the available evidence concluded that no significant difference with regard to clinical, ongoing pregnancy rates and live birth rates were found comparing true NC-FET to HRT-FET (33). However the conclusion of this meta-analysis should not be universally accepted without determining the methods adopted in each study to determine the timing of ovulation which we know is of critical importance. Only two studies included in this meta-analysis used serum samples to identify the LH surge (34, 35) and the study by Xiao et al., used urinary LH tests for LH surge identification (36). Due to the aforementioned possible inaccuracies of urinary LH detection kits, the findings of this study are questionable.

Recently published studies comparing NC-FET to other approaches for endometrial preparation used solely ultrasonographic disappearance of the dominant follicle in combination with urinary LH tests for detection of ovulation (37, 38). The outcomes are contradictory as the study by Cardenas et al. (37) favored NC-FET whereas Madani et al. (38) did not find one approach superior to the other.

9.3 Pitfalls to Consider When Interpreting Study Conclusions

The critical step in a HRT-FET cycle is to adjust the duration of progesterone exposure to the developmental stage of the embryo following estradiol administration to prepare the endometrium. The route and duration of progesterone exposure has to be critically appraised in studies comparing the outcome of embryo transfer regimens as they may pose pitfalls in the correct timing of embryo transfer.

Different routes of progesterone administration as well as different durations of progesterone exposure pose a possible bias as seen in the study of Devine et al. (39). This study evaluated the efficacy of vaginal progesterone administration, either alone or in combination with intramuscular progesterone every third day, compared to daily intramuscular progesterone in terms of pregnancy and live birth rates following transfers of vitrified-warmed blastocysts and published the data of the interim analysis. The authors concluded that the vaginal only protocol is inferior to the approach which includes i.m. progesterone administration. It has to be noted that in the study group which received intramuscular progesterone only, the endometrium was exposed to progesterone one-half day longer as compared to the groups receiving either vaginal progesterone or the combination of vaginal and i.m. progesterone. The different exposure times of the endometrium to progesterone and the different administration routes have to be taken into account in this study rendering it impossible to concur with the author's conclusion.

Recently, two high impact factor journals published multicenter trials which compared fresh ET and NC-FET (40) and fresh ET versus NC-FET and HRT-FET (41), respectively. The studies came to contradictory conclusions, with Shi et al. (40) reporting no difference in the livebirth rate between fresh and frozen ET among ovulatory women with infertility and Wei et al. (41) finding a higher singleton livebirth rate in FET compared to fresh ET. These contradictory findings may be explained by suboptimal methodology in the timing of embryo transfer in the natural FET cycles. Both studies based the identification of ovulation and timing of the subsequent embryo transfer purely on ultrasound scan findings with no detailed description of the ultrasound criteria used to define ovulation. We can only assume that the disappearance of the dominant follicle was used as the criteria to define ovulation. The issue with using ultrasound confirmation of dominant follicle disappearance as the sole criteria for defining "ovulation" lies in the fact that different patterns of follicular fluid evacuation during ovulation have been described. It is important to note, that in some cases fluid remains in the former follicle even into the luteal phase (42). Therefore, ultrasonographic detection of dominant follicle disappearance is not reliable in isolation to precisely identify ovulation and will result in inaccurate timing of embryo transfer.

Ovulation detection by a combination of ultrasound monitoring of follicular growth and serial measurement of LH, estradiol, and progesterone levels is recognized to be the most accurate method of correctly identifying ovulation (43). This is the optimal method of determining accurately the time of ovulation and is the method which should be adopted in scientific studies of the natural cycle.

9.4 Conclusions

Synchrony of the endometrium and the embryo developmental stage is crucial for implantation in FET, in both natural and HRT cycles. As endometrial receptivity is closely correlated to the time of progesterone exposure following sufficient estrogen exposure, timing of the embryo transfer is the key step toward a successful outcome in addition to embryo euploidy and embryo quality. The conclusions of previous studies, comparing the outcome of different approaches to endometrial preparation for FET have to be critically evaluated for the "correct" timing of the embryo transfer. Further large prospective randomized studies comparing HRT-FET to correctly conducted natural cycles for FET are required to determine the optimal cycle regimen.

References

1. Niederberger C, Pellicer A, Cohen J, et al. Forty years of IVF. Fertil Steril 2018;110 (2):185–324.

2. Loutradi KE, Kolibianakis EM, Venetis CA, et al. Cryopreservation of human embryos by vitrification or slow freezing: a systematic review and meta-analysis. Fertil Steril 2008;90(1):186–193.

3. Le Lannou D, Griveau JF, Laurent MC, et al. Contribution of embryo cryopreservation to elective single embryo transfer in IVF-ICSI. Reprod Biomed Online 2006;13:368–375.

4. Ethics Committee of the American Society for Reproductive Medicine. Fertility preservation and reproduction in cancer patients. Fertil Steril 2005;83:1622–1628.

5. Ethics Committee of the American Society for Reproductive Medicine. Planned oocyte cryopreservation for women seeking to preserve future reproductive potential: an Ethics Committee opinion. Fertil Steril 2018;110 (6):1022–1028.

6. Dahdouh EM, Balayla J, García Velasco JA. Comprehensive chromosome screening improves embryo selection: a meta-analysis. Fertil Steril 2015;104(6):1503–1512.

7. Navot D, Scott RT, Droesch K, et al. The window of embryo transfer and the efficiency of human conception in vitro. Fertil Steril 1991;55:114–118.

8. Harper MJK. The implantation window. Baillieres Clin Obstet Gynaecol 1992;6:351–371.

9. Giudice LC. Potential biochemical markers of uterine receptivity. Hum Reprod 1999;14(Suppl 2):3–16.

10. Hoozemans DA, Schats R, Lambalk CB, et al. Human embryo implantation: current knowledge and clinical implications in assisted reproductive technology. Reprod Biomed Online 2004;9:692–715.

11. Kodaman P, Taylor H. Hormonal regulation of implantation. Obstet Gynecol Clin N Am 2004;31:745–766.

12. Noyes RW, Hertig AT, Rock J. Dating the endometrial biopsy. Fertil Steril 1950;1:561–564.

13. Christenson LK, Devoto L. Cholesterol transport and steroidogenesis by the corpus luteum. Reprod Biol Endocrinol 2003;1:90.

14. Devoto L, Fuentes A, Kohen P, et al. The human corpus luteum: life cycle and function in natural cycles. Fertil Steril 2009;92:1067–1079.

15. Loke YW, King A, Burrows TD. Decidua in human implantation. Hum Reprod 1995;10(Suppl 2):14–21.

16. Psychoyos A. Uterine receptivity for nidation. Ann N Y Acad Sci 1986;476:36–42.

17. Psychoyos A. Hormonal control of ovoimplantation. Vitam Horm 1973;31:201–256.

18. Testart J, Frydman R, Feinstein MC, et al. Interpretation of plasma luteinizing hormone assay for the collection of mature oocytes from women: definition of a luteinizing hormone surge-initiating rise. Fertil Steril 1981;36(1):50–54.

19. Frydman R, Testart J, Feinstein MC, et al. Interrelationship of plasma and urinary luteinizing hormone preovulatory surge. J Steroid Biochem 1984;20:617–619.

20. Miller PB, Soules MR. The usefulness of urinary LH kit for ovulation prediction during menstrual cycles of normal women. Obstet Gynecol 1996;87:13–17.

21. Krotz S, McKenzie LJ, Cisneros P, et al. Prevalence of premature urinary luteinizing hormone surges in women with regular menstrual cycles and its effect on implantation of frozen-thawed embryos. Fertil Steril 2005;83 (6):1742–1744.

22. www.hfea.gov.uk/media/2563/hfea-fertility-trends-and-figures-2017-v2.pdf.

23. de Wit H, Schmitt L, Purdy R, et al. Effects of acute progesterone administration in healthy postmenopausal women and normally-cycling women. Psychoneuroendocrinology 2001;26 (7):697–710.

24. Myers ER, Sondheimer SJ, Freeman EW, et al. Serum progesterone levels following vaginal administration of progesterone during the luteal phase. Fertil Steril 1987;47 (1):71–75.

25. Villanueva B, Casper RF, Yen SS. Intravaginal administration of progesterone: enhanced absorption after estrogen treatment. Fertil Steril 1981;35:433–437.

26. Fatemi HM, Kyrou D, Bourgain C, et al. Cryopreserved-thawed human embryo transfer: spontaneous natural cycle is superior to human chorionic gonadotropin-induced natural cycle. Fertil Steril 2010;94(6):2054–2058.

27. Zimmermann G, Ackermann W, Alexander H. Epithelial human chorionic gonadotropin is expressed and produced in human secretory endometrium during the normal menstrual cycle. Biol Reprod 2009;80:1053–1065.

28. Ghobara T, Vandekerckhove P. Cycle regimens for frozen-thawed embryo transfer. Cochrane Database Syst Rev 2008;23(1):CD003414.

29. Ghobara T, Gelbaya TA, Ayeleke RO. Cycle regimens for frozen-thawed embryo transfer. Cochrane Database Syst Rev 2017;7(7):CD003414.

30. Cattoli M, Ciotti PM, Seracchioli R, et al. A randomized prospective study on cryopreserved-thawed embryo transfer: natural versus hormone replacement cycles. In: *10th Annual Meeting of the ESHRE, Brussels*. Vol. 356. ESHRE, 1994:139.

31. Karimzadeh MA, Mohammadian F, Mashayekhy M. Comparison of frozen-thawed embryo transfer outcome in natural cycle and hormone replacement cycle. Hum Reprod 2012;27(Suppl 2):284.

32. Groenewoud ER, Cohlen B, Al-Oraiby A, et al. A randomized controlled non-inferiority trial of modified natural versus artificial cycle for cryo-thawed embryo transfer. Hum Reprod 2016;31 (7):1483–1492.

33. Groenewoud ER, Cantineau AE, Kollen BJ, et al. What is the optimal means of preparing the endometrium in frozen-thawed embryo transfer cycles? A systematic review and meta-analysis. Hum Reprod Update 2017;23(2):255–261.

34. Morozov V, Ruman J, Kenigsberg D, et al. Natural cycle cryo-thaw transfer may improve pregnancy outcome. J Assist Reprod Genet 2007;24:119–123.

35. Chang EM, Han JE, Kim YS, et al. Use of the natural cycle and vitrification thawed

blastocyst transfer results in better in-vitro fertilization outcomes: cycle regimens of vitrification thawed blastocyst transfer. J Assist Reprod Genet 2011;28 369–374.

36. Xiao Z, Zhou X, Xu W, et al. Natural cycle is superior to hormone replacement therapy cycle for vitrificated – preserved frozen-thawed embryo transfer. Syst Biol Reprod Med 2011;58:107–112.

37. Cardenas Armas DF, Peñarrubia J, Goday A, et al. Frozen-thawed blastocyst transfer in natural cycle increase implantation rates compared artificial cycle. Gynecol Endocrinol 2019;11:1–5.

38. Madani T, Ramezanali F, Yahyaei A, et al. Live birth rates after different endometrial preparation methods in frozen cleavage-stage embryo transfer cycles: a randomized controlled trial. Arch Gynecol Obstet 2019;299(4):1185–1191.

39. Devine K, Richter KS, Widra EA, et al. Vitrified blastocyst transfer cycles with the use of only vaginal progesterone replacement with Endometrin have inferior ongoing pregnancy rates: results from the planned interim analysis of a three-arm randomized controlled noninferiority trial. Fertil Steril 2018;109 (2):266–275.

40. Shi Y, Sun Y, Hao C, et al. Transfer of fresh versus frozen embryos in ovulatory women. N Engl J Med 2018;378 (2):126–136.

41. Wei D, Liu J-Y, Sun Y, et al. Frozen versus fresh single blastocyst transfer in ovulatory women: a multicentre, randomised controlled trial. Lancet 2019;393:1310–1318.

42. Hanna MD, Chizen DR, Pierson RA. Characteristics of follicular evacuation during human ovulation. Ultrasound Obstet Gynecol 1994;4 (6):488–493.

43. Irani M, Robles A, Gunnala V, et al. Optimal parameters for determining the LH surge in natural cycle frozen-thawed embryo transfers. J Ovarian Res 2017;10(1):70.

Individualized Immunological Testing in Recurrent Implantation Failure

Diana Alecsandru and Juan Antonio García Velasco

10.1 Introduction

Human reproduction is an inefficient process. Still today is no clear definition for recurrent implantation failure (RIF). It is a condition arising from the failure of a successive number of in vitro fertilization cycles (IVF) in which theoretically the pregnancy should have already been achieved. Due to the disparity in the implantation and pregnancy rates among different assisted reproduction centers, a consensus definition has not been achieved. Technological and scientific advances in the field of ART have led to better reproductive outcomes. Despite all the efforts, around 30 percent of healthy euploid embryos still fail to implant today (1).

Disruptions in maternal immune tolerance have been invoked as one cause of implantation failure. The original theory was that immunosuppression was required to tolerate the presence of the allogeneic fetus. Owing to repeated failed cycles even after gamete donation, we all have witnessed increasing patient demand for immune tests and "immune treatments."

The role of the immune system in recurrent miscarriage (RM) and recurrent implantation failure (RIF) is one of the most controversial issues in ART (2). Controversy is partly due to the fact that most studies of the immune system in reproduction have focused on finding markers of peripheral blood mostly based on the number or percentage of specific immune cells (3, 4) and on the use of immunosuppression (5, 6). The main reason why immune treatments have failed so far, and why immune tests (peripheral blood natural killer [pbNK] or uterine natural killer [uNK] cell testing) have shown very weak or no predictive values, is basically poor study design and great patient heterogeneity (7).

Immune system cells have an important role in immune defense and reproduction. Natural killer (NK) cells have become a central element in immunological studies for women suffering recurrent miscarriage (RM) and recurrent implantation failure (RIF). They specialize in killing virus-infected and tumor-transformed target cells by the balanced action of both activating and inhibitory receptors (8). Several studies have tagged NK cells as killers in charge of rejecting the embryo, and have associated this function with reproductive failure (4).

Uterine NK cells (uNK) are phenotypically distinct from those circulating in blood; they are CD56^{bright}, CD16- whereas 90 percent of blood NK cells are CD56^{dim}, CD16+ (9). The minor CD56^{bright} population in blood also differ from those in the uterus morphologically and for many other surface markers. These differences mean that measurements of any NK parameters in NK cells from blood will not be informative in relation to function of uNK (5).

Uterine NK cells proliferate and differentiate in the mucosa. They are not present premenarche or postmenopausally and their dependence on the ovarian hormone, progesterone, is obvious from the great surge in proliferative activity after ovulation. This is mediated by increased expression of IL-15 from stromal cells in response to progesterone. The presence of uNK in the decidua is maximal in the first trimester and numbers thereafter fall so although they are still present at term they are not abundant (10).

Killer immunoglobulin-like receptors (KIRs) determine the NK cell function in the context of other receptor-ligand interactions and permutations of 28 NK cell receptors, which result in at least 10,000 different NK cell subsets in a given individual (11). Furthermore, the KIR repertoires of uNK and pbNK differ when taken from the same woman at the same time.

The activity of the uterine NK cells, $CD56^{bright}CD16-$, is influenced by the KIR repertoires, and differ absolutely from pbNKs in phenotype markers and functional activity (12). The uNK killing function is very weak compared with pbNK. With infections, this can change as the CMV infection elicits a different uNK effector function. uNK cells are capable of controlling cytomegalovirus (CMV) infection and acquiring the cytotoxic phenotype against CMV-infected decidual fibroblasts by means of receptor repertoire modulation (13), but this process has not been shown against a healthy embryo.

The number and function of pbNK and uNK cells show wide variability depending on the patient's clinical condition, e.g., infections, autoimmunity, or tumor or the day of menstrual cycle. Studies of NK cells and reproductive issues have not taken this NK cell physiologic variation into account, nor differences in pbNK and uNK cell receptors, whose activation is essential for its functions.

Thus, the increased number of uNKs in the secretory phase of the normal menstrual cycle and pregnancy (90 percent of local immune cells in the first trimester of pregnancy) is a physiologic process that focuses on helping embryo implantation and is not a marker of "embryo rejection."

However, this physiological maternal–fetal immune tolerance could be imbalanced with a negative impact over embryo implantation and placentation. The maternal–fetal tolerance failure, a tissue-restricted process, does not have a systemic impact on the peripheral immune cells and tests based on the percentage or number of peripheral blood immune cells, Th1 cytokine, or NK cytotoxicity assays did not reflect the immune endometrial imbalance.

The expression of maternal immune system dysregulation could be

1. a lack of activation with negative signals into the maternal–fetal tolerance and impaired embryo implantation or placentation
2. an over reactivity with an increased inflammatory uterine environment and damage on the trophoblast cells

10.2 Maternal Adaptation to the Fetus

Successful maternal adaptation to the semiallogenic fetus occurs in the uterus at the site of placentation. The key of materno-fetal tolerance process is the remodeling of the spiral arteries, with destruction of the media by invading extravillous trophoblast (EVT) cells.

Most immune cells in the endometrium are tissue-resident cells and their number, type, and activation state are highly dependent on the hormonal environment. Maternal uterine immune cells actively respond to fetal antigens, promoting maternal–fetal immune tolerance as observed in a normal pregnancy. Uterine NK cells (uNK) regulate trophoblast invasion and enhance vascular remodeling by extravillous trophoblast (11) and Treg cells (FoxP3+Treg), promoting maternal–fetal immune tolerance. Human trophoblasts express a battery of immune inhibitory molecules predominantly targeting T cells (CD4+ or CD8+), such as Fas ligand or indoleamine 2,3-dioxygenase (IDO), which are potent inducers of T cell apoptosis as a protective mechanism of maternal–fetal tolerance. The interaction between trophoblast HLA-G dimers and LILRB1 receptors expressed by macrophage and dendritic cells also promotes maternal–fetal tolerance.

In terms of allorecognition, interactions between members of the killer immunoglobulin-like receptor (KIR) family expressed by uNK cells binding to trophoblast HLA-C molecules are of particular interest, as both maternal KIR and fetal HLA-C genes are highly polymorphic. This means that there will be different maternal/fetal genetic combinations in each pregnancy. The variability in the KIR gene family is both at the level of presence/absence of a gene and the individual allelic variability at each KIR locus.

Placentation is regulated by interactions between maternal KIRs expressed by uNKs, and fetal HLA-C molecules, expressed by EVTs. Hiby et al. (14) showed that invading EVTs are the principal site of HLA-C expression in the decidua basalis and that both maternal and paternal HLA-C allotypes are presented to KIRs. Insufficient invasion of the uterine lining by trophoblasts and vascular conversion in the decidua are thought to be the primary defect in disorders such as recurrent miscarriages (RM), preeclampsia, and fetal growth restriction (FGR).

Several studies conducted in natural pregnancies by Hiby and Moffett (15) showed that women who have a KIR AA genotype (two KIR A haplotypes) are at risk of preeclampsia and other pregnancy disorders when the fetus has more HLA-C2 genes than the mother and when additional fetal HLA-C2 alleles are of paternal origin.

Also, they described that protection from preeclampsia is likely mediated by activating KIR2DS1 (B haplotype), which also binds HLA-C2. Thus, depending on the particular KIR–HLA-C interaction, trophoblast cell invasion is regulated.

Assisted pregnancies differ from medically unassisted pregnancies. These patients receive sometimes more than one embryo per transfer, and also donor oocytes, sperm donor or embryo donation, are often used. After double embryo transfer (DET), the expression of more than one paternal HLA-C per trophoblast cell is induced. In oocyte donation cycles, an increasingly demanded treatment due to advanced maternal age, the oocyte-maternal HLA-C, which is genetically different from the mother's receptor, behaves as a paternal HLA-C and this induces that more nonself HLA antigens are presented to the mother's KIR (per transfer) compared with "normal" pregnancies.

When donor oocytes or embryos are used, the embryo shares no maternal "self" genes, as both sets of chromosomes are derived from "nonself" individuals. In other words, the oocyte HLA-C allele is genetically different from the surrogate mother's HLA-C alleles, and thus the oocyte HLA-C allele represents an additional "paternal" or nonself HLA-C, increasing the number of foreign HLA-C alleles to be faced by the mother immune uterine cells.

Previous research has highlighted the risk for women and their babies in oocyte donation pregnancies. Consistent findings are the increased risk of pregnancy-induced hypertension and other great obstetrical syndromes (preeclampsia and fetal growth restriction, FGR), even when controlling for age and singleton pregnancies.

For the first time in 2014 (16), our group reported a significantly decreased LBR per cycle after a DET with donated oocytes in KIR AA patients when compared to KIR AB and KIR BB.

The increased expression of paternal HLA-C after DET is associated with more pregnancy disorders than single embryo transfer (SET) in mothers with an inhibitory KIR haplotype (AA).

The decreased LBR after DET in donor oocyte cycles in mothers KIR AA may be due to increased expression of nonself HLA-C (paternal and oocyte donor HLA-C). In this case 4 "paternal" HLA-C per trophoblast cells/DET: 1 paternal and 1 oocyte donor HLA-C per trophoblast cell and embryo since oocyte donor HLA-C behaves as "paternal" nonself HLA-C. Expressing 4 "paternal" HLA-C is more likely to find at least one paternal or oocyte donor HLA-C2 than in own oocytes and SET, and probably implantation or placentation failure occurs in mothers who are KIR AA.

This new findings show that the maternal KIR haplotype and fetal HLA-C have an impact on the live birth rate after IVF cycles, especially when donor oocyte and DET are used. Expressing four paternal HLA-C in the EVT cells after DET with donor oocytes is more likely to result in at least one nonself HLA-C2 (even by HLA-C2 allelic frequency on Caucasian population) than with one's own oocyte after SET, and implantation or placentation failure probably occurs in mothers with the KIR AA haplotype. Therefore, selecting HLA-C1 among oocyte and/or sperm donors for patients undergoing egg donation and inhibitory KIR haplotypes could be more efficient and safer (17).

The combination of maternal KIR haplotype and parental, donors HLA-C, could predict which couple can benefit for the selection of SET/DET, or donor selection by HLA-C in ART, in order to increase the LBR/cycle and it would facilitate the reduction of embryos that are being transferred, facilitating the increase of SET with an impact over pregnancy complication (preeclampsia, FGR, etc.) too. Therefore, selecting HLA-C1 among oocyte and/or sperm donors for patients undergoing to egg donation ART and inhibitory KIR, could be more efficient and safer as identified by epidemiological studies (15, 19, 20) (see also Figures 10.1 and 10.2).

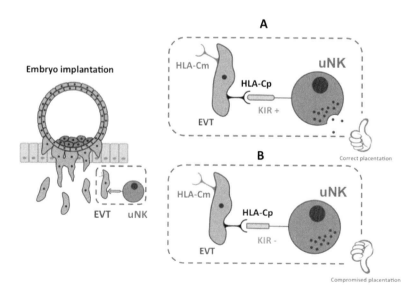

Figure 10.1 Maternal–fetal immune recognition in own oocytes single embryo transfer. (A) Correct activation through maternal KIR with a matched fetal HLA-C. (B) Inhibitory KIR signals after a contact with a mismatch fetal HLA-C. A black and white version of this figure will appear in some formats. For the colour version, please refer to the plate section.

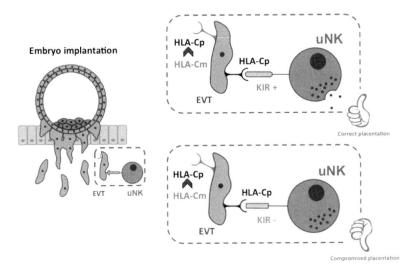

Figure 10.2 An egg donor embryo. The "maternal" HLA-C behaves as paternal, since, from a genetic point of view, it's foreign for the mother. So, in this case, the egg donor's HLA-C also needs to find the right receptor to induce good placentation. A black and white version of this figure will appear in some formats. For the colour version, please refer to the plate section.

10.3 Maternal Immune System Overreactivity

Autoimmune connective tissue diseases (e.g., rheumatoid arthritis, systemic lupus erythematosus, antiphospholipid antibody syndrome, systemic sclerosis, primary Sjogren's syndrome, inflammatory myositis) predominantly affect women (9 : 1 ratio to males) and often occur during the reproductive years and their debut or activity can have a negative impact on reproductive outcomes (21, 22). The planning of the embryo transfer according to the clinical stability of the autoimmune disease could minimize the pregnancy risks. An emphasis on preconception counseling and strict disease control in the months prior to conception are essential components of this new era of pregnancy, ART, and autoimmune diseases (23).

10.4 Antiphospholipid (aPL) Syndrome (APS)

The antiphospholipid (aPL) syndrome (APS) is an acquired autoimmune thrombophilic condition that is a cause of pregnancy complications attributable to placental insufficiency including recurrent pregnancy loss, IUGR, oligohydramnios, preeclampsia, and placental abruption.

Patients with APS do not have a higher infertility rate than the general population. However, they have worse reproductive results and a higher risk of gestational complications. Studies on the impact of aPL antibodies (antiPL Abs) and the results of ART suffer from multiple methodological limitations and therefore, the detrimental impact of aPL Abs positivity is controversial. The vast majority of studies investigating an association between antiPL Abs and infertility use arbitrary cutoff levels that do not respect diagnostic consensus. Few studies have included the β2-glycoprotein I Abs and none has confirmed the positivity after 12 weeks (24). The published results are thus contradictory. Some studies found association between positivity of aPL Abs and RIF but others, did not (25).

Currently the study of aPL Abs in patients with RIF should be clinically individualized, as there is no clear recommendation for or against their analysis.

Celiac disease (CD) is nowadays recognized as an immune-mediated systemic disease related to dietary gluten ingestion in genetically susceptible children and adults. It is associated to a variety of symptoms, intestinal and extraintestinal, being common mild symptoms or even subclinical disease. Development of noninvasive serological tests for diagnosis prompted to develop screening programs in those groups with increased risk for CD, such as first degree relatives of CD patients or people with certain symptoms or disorders. The association between infertility and autoimmune diseases has long been recognized. Related to CD, undiagnosed disease can be associated to recurrent spontaneous abortions, intrauterine growth restriction, low birth weight, delayed menarche, early menopause. Therefore, serological testing in women with reproductive problems could help to identify undetected CD cases.

Including infertility in the group of CD associated conditions caused a big controversy, and a consensus has not been reached due to the contradictory results found in the literature.

Despite the increasing number of papers relating CD and adverse pregnancy outcomes, there is not unanimous consensus about considering women with reproductive problems as a risk group for CD. We reported recently better reproductive outcome under gluten free diet in celiac patients compared to normal diet (26).

In an exploratory study, several serological tests were used to select patients with potential CD and to identify who requires an intestinal biopsy to diagnose CD. Following current guidelines, IgA anti-TG2 was determined as the first line test for CD screening.

Current knowledge does not allow giving specific recommendations about general screening of CD in women with recurrent reproductive failure. Similarly to the general population, 1 percent CD prevalence should be probably expected when performing anti-TG2-based serological screening, but additionally a similar percentage of undetected cases could exist. Further studies are still needed, preferentially with a prospective design and careful handling of the beneficial effect of the GFD on reproductive outcomes.

10.5 Metabolic and Autoimmune Disorders

In the last decade, mean age of infertile women undergoing ART has increased. Age is one of the main risk factors for disorders like functional glucose impairment or hypertension. In the clinical work-up of the patients, only fasting glucose levels are included among metabolic tests.

During ART, the "silent" metabolic disorders and their impact over reproductive outcome has been less studied.

Women suffering from recurrent implantation failure (RIF) or recurrent miscarriage (RM) may undergo different tests trying to understand their poor reproductive outcome. Metabolic routine screening for all infertile patients is not recommended, but a tailored approach may be needed for some subsets of patients that could improve their reproductive outcome.

Diabetes is a complex disease and the classification into Type 1 and Type 2 does not include all metabolic disorders related with impaired insulin secretion or action. Type 1 diabetes is an autoimmune disease characterized by immunological pancreatic attack by autoreactive T cells and auto-antibodies with severe loss of insulin secretion. Around

5–14 percent of patients classified with Type 2 diabetes have diabetes-associated autoanti-bodies. The term latent autoimmune diabetes in adults (LADA) has been introduced for this autoimmune diabetes characterized by adult onset, presence of diabetes-associated auto-antibodies, and more frequent need for insulin treatment than patients with classical Type 2 diabetes. LADA is the most prevalent form of adult-onset autoimmune diabetes and probably the most prevalent form of autoimmune diabetes in general. A high frequency of thyroid and gastric autoimmunity among LADA patients and positive HLA-DR3 and DR4 has been described showing a genetic association among autoimmune endocrine diseases. In reproductive field, most of the tests to detect functional glucose impairment are used during pregnancy and less is known about its usefulness in the preconception period even more in assisted reproductive treatment (ART).

A recent study (27) observed a significantly increased live birth rates (LBR) per cycle (52 percent) after a precise diagnosis and adequate metabolic status compared with LBR/cycle without pancreatic autoimmunity control (7.5 percent) ($p < 0.0001$).

The diabetes-associated autoantibodies (DAA) appear even years before LADA diag-nosis. The current preconceptional protocols do not include tests to detect pancreatic autoimmunity and affected women presenting RIF or RM are often misdiagnosed. Before the embryo transfer (ET) the routine tests include only fasting plasma glucose and a normal level is considered as normal metabolic function. Immune or metabolic routine screening for all infertile couples is not advised but a tailored approach is useful for some subsets of patients having "silent" immune or metabolic disorders.

Anti-GAD Antibodies (Abs) can be detected years before the clinical onset of auto-immunediabetes, which indicate a long prediabetes autoimmune period.

Anti-GAD positivity is associated with high-risk HLA haplotypes linked to type 1 DM and also thyroid autoimmunity.

For glycemic disorders only fasting glucose is tested before starting ART and this determination falls short in some subset of patients. Recently, it has been recommended to perform in obese women, in lean PCOS women with advanced age (>40 years), as well as in the presence of a personal history of gestational diabetes or family history of type 2 DM, but few details are known about the autoimmune diabetes among reproductive-age and -risk population. In our subset of patients (27) (2.7 percent of our RM and RIF cohort) we have observed that patients affected by autoimmune pancreatic disorders, using the routine tests and having normal BMI, HbA1 c, and fasting glucose and insulin levels, could be considered as having a normal metabolic state before ART. But, 85 percent of them have thyroid autoimmune disease associated with family history of DM (100 percent) and it is known that the autoimmune thyroid disease and autoimmune diabetes frequently occur in the same individual because of a strong shared genetic susceptibility. We reported (26) that patients with RM or RIF of unknown etiology diagnosed with thyroid autoimmune dis-orders, family history of diabetes, and impaired insulin response after OGTT could be considered as a subset of patients, candidates for further specific autoimmune tests to rule out DAA.

In patients with family history of DM, the OGTT could help to detect the insulin secretion impairment even more if those patients have other autoimmune disease.

The incidence of pancreatic autoimmunity or LADA among women undergoing to ART is unknown and probably is not so high (2.7 percent in our RM and RIF cohort); but is quite easy, by clinical and metabolic characteristics described, to identify this subset of patients and recommend a correct treatment with a positive impact in their preconception management and reproductive result after ET.

10.6 Conclusions

A maternal immune system dysregulation could have a negative impact on the embryo implantation and placentation.

The maternal immune system imbalance can be summarized as

1. a lack of activation with negative signals into the maternal–fetal tolerance and impaired embryo implantation or placentation
2, an overreactivity with an increased inflammatory uterine environment and damage on the trophoblast cells

According to these clinical scenarios, the immune tests useful in patients with RIF are

* KIR and HLA-C
* autoimmunity: a clinically individualized immune tests for celiac disease screening, metabolic issues, or specific autoimmune disorders in a multidisciplinary specialized unit

References

1. Franasiak JM, Scott RT. Contribution of immunology to implantation failure of euploid embryos. Fertil Steril 2017;107:1279–1283.

2. Alecsandru D, García-Velasco JA. Immune testing and treatment: still an open debate. Hum Reprod 2015;30:1994.

3. Sacks G. Enough! Stop the arguments and get on with the science of naturalkiller cell testing. Hum Reprod 2015;30:1526–1531.

4. Tang AW, Alfirevic Z, Quenby S. Natural killer cells and pregnancy outcomes in women with recurrent miscarriage and infertility: a systematic review. Hum Reprod 2011;26:1971–1980.

5. Moffett A, Shreeve N. Reply: First do no harm: continuing the uterine NK celldebate. Hum Reprod 2015;31:218–219.

6. Moffett A, Shreeve N. First do no harm: uterine natural killer (NK) cells in assisted reproduction. Hum Reprod 2015;30:1519–1525.

7. Alecsandru D, García-Velasco JA. Immunology and human reproduction. Curr Opin Obstet Gynecol 2015;27:231–234.

8. Farag SS, Caligiuri MA. Human natural killer cell development and biology. Blood Rev 2006;20:123–137.

9. Moffett A, Chazara O, Colucci F. Maternal allo-recognition of the fetus. Fertil Steril 2017;107:1269–1272.

10. Trundley A, Moffett A. Human uterine leukocytes and pregnancy. Tissue Antigens 2004;63:1–12.

11. Moffett A, Colucci F. Co-evolution of NK receptors and HLA ligands in humans is driven by reproduction. Immunol Rev 2015;267:283–297.

12. Koopman LA, Kopcow HD, Rybalov B, et al. Human decidual natural killer cells are a unique NK cell subset with immunomodulatory potential. J Exp Med 2003;198:1201–1212.

13. Siewiera J, El Costa H, Tabiasco J, et al. Human cytomegalovirus infection elicits new decidual natural killer cell effector functions. PLoS Pathog 2013;9:e1003257.

14. Hiby SE, Regan L, Lo W, et al. Association of maternal killer-cell immunoglobulin-like receptors and parental HLA-C genotypes with recurrent miscarriage. Hum Reprod 2008;23:972–976.

15. Hiby SE, Apps R, Sharkey AM, et al. Maternal activating KIRs protect against human reproductive failure mediated by fetal HLA-C2. J Clin Invest 2010;120:4102–4110.

16. Alecsandru D, Garrido N, Vicario JL, et al. Maternal KIR haplotype influences live birth rate after double embryo transfer in IVF cycles in patients with recurrent miscarriages and implantation failure. Hum Reprod 2014;29:2637–2643.

17. Alecsandru D, García-Velasco JA. Why natural killer cells are not enough: a further understanding of killer immunoglobulin-like receptor and human leukocyte antigen. Fertil Steril 2017;107:1273–1278.

18. Moffett A, Colucci F. Uterine NK cells: active regulators at the maternal-fetalinterface. J Clin Invest 2014;124:1872–1879.

19. Skjaerven R, Vatten LJ, Wilcox AJ, et al. Recurrence of pre-eclampsia across generations: exploring fetal and maternal genetic components in a population based cohort. BMJ 2005;331:877.

20. Marder W, Littlejohn EA, Somers EC. Pregnancy and autoimmune connective tissue diseases. Best Pract Res Clin Rheumatol 2016;30(1):63–80.

21. Lambert M, Hocké C, Jimenez C, et al. Repeated in vitro fertilization failure: Abnormalities identified in the diagnostic assessment. Gynecol Obstet Fertil 2016;44 (10):565–571.

22. Andreoli L. EULAR recommendations for women's health and the management of family planning, assisted reproduction, pregnancy and menopause in patients with systemic lupus erythematosus and/or antiphospholipid syndrome. Ann Rheum Dis. 2017;76 (3):476–485.

23. Khizroeva J, Makatsariya A, Bitsadze V, et al. In vitro fertilization outcomes in women with antiphospholipid antibodies circulation. J Matern Fetal Neonatal Med 2018;33:1–11.

24. Ata B, Urman B. Thrombophilia and assisted reproduction technology-any detrimental impact or unnecessary overuse? J Assist Reprod Genet 2016;33:1305–1310.

25. Alecsandru D, López-Palacios N, Mercedes C, et al. Exploring undiagnosed celiac disease in women with recurrent reproductive failure: reproductive outcomes could improve with a gluten free diet. Am J Reprod Immunol 2019;10: e13209.

26. Alecsandru D, Barrio A, Andia V, et al. Pancreatic autoimmunity: an unknown etiology on patients with assisted reproductive techniques (ART)-recurrent reproductive failure. PLoS One 2018;13 (10):e0203446.

27. Parental human leukocyte antigen-C allotypes are predictive of live birth rate and risk of poor placentation in assisted reproductive treatment. Alecsandru D, Barrio A, Garrido N, Aparicio P, Pellicer A, Moffett A, García-Velasco JA. Fertil Steril. 2020 Jul 30:S0015-0282(20)30443-X

Individualized Embryo Transfer

Carol Coughlan, Luisa Loiudice, and Antonio Pellicer

11.1 Introduction

Despite the various advances and the increasing success rates of assisted conception treatment, implantation continues to be a rate limiting step. For implantation to occur a blastocyst must attach to and invade the endometrium and as such both the embryo and endometrium are considered critical to the process of implantation. However, there are other factors to consider. Many conditions of the uterine cavity may influence the ability of the embryo to implant such as uterine submucosal fibroids and endometrial polyps, which are well recognized to exert an adverse effect. In addition, an embryo's implantation potential may be affected by sperm and oocyte quality. Iatrogenic factors such as laboratory conditions and embryo transfer technique play an important role in successful implantation, hence this chapter will focus on the embryo transfer procedure. This is the final step in the treatment cycle, the culmination of both clinicians' and embryologists' efforts and a day of great hope for the patients. The importance of the embryo transfer procedure is not to be underestimated. This chapter will highlight the importance to clinicians of not adopting a "one-size-fits-all" approach when planning embryo transfer. It is incumbent on reproductive medicine specialists to focus on the embryo transfer procedure, try to preempt any potential issues that may adversely affect success rates and adopt an individualized plan for embryo transfer when necessary.

11.2 To Transfer in Fresh or Frozen Cycles?

In recent years, the number of frozen-thawed embryo transfer (FET) cycles performed has increased significantly facilitated by improved laboratory techniques. Embryo cryopreservation has undoubtedly resulted in increased IVF/ICSI cycle cumulative pregnancy rates.

A factor contributing to the increasing incidence of elective embryo cryopreservation has been the accumulating evidence to suggest that IVF outcomes may be improved by performing FET cycles as compared to fresh embryo transfers (1, 2). Studies have suggested that controlled ovarian hyperstimulation adversely affects endometrial receptivity (3–5). Kolibianakis et al. demonstrated that endometrial advancement on the day of oocyte retrieval is present in all cycles stimulated with GnRH antagonists, recombinant FSH and hCG (5). The chance of pregnancy is significantly decreased in the presence of extreme endometrial advancement at the time of oocyte retrieval (5). This adverse affect of ovarian stimulation on endometrial receptivity is attributed to supraphysiological levels of both estrogen and progesterone inducing morphological and biochemical endometrial alterations resulting in a more advanced endometrium as compared to natural cycles (6–8). This endometrial advancement leads to asynchrony between embryo stage and endometrium which may be avoided by preferentially cryopreserving embryos and transferring them later into a more physiologically normal environment (6–8). Studies also suggest that super-ovulation may be detrimental to implantation by altering genes crucial for the endometrium–embryo interaction (9, 10). Many studies have suggested a freeze-all policy in which all embryos are electively cryopreserved for transfer in a subsequent frozen-thaw cycle in the hopes of providing a more physiological environment for embryo transfer and improving implantation and pregnancy rates (11–13).

For patients who experience repeated implantation failure despite the transfer of good-quality embryos, preimplantation genetic screening and elective "freeze-all" should be considered and discussed with the couple. It is interesting to note that a recent prospective cohort study identified a statistically significant improvement in ongoing pregnancy and implantation rates following a freeze-all policy for patients with recurrent implantation failure (14).

For patients planning preimplantation genetic screening, cryopreservation of embryos facilitates trophectoderm biopsy. The current testing method of blastocyst-stage trophectoderm biopsy with the use of next-generation sequencing (NGS) and 24 chromosome screening has resulted in significantly improved implantation rates as compared to the initial day 3 single blastomere biopsy and the initial genetic testing method FISH (fluorescence in situ hybridization).

Undoubtedly, ovarian stimulation with exogenous gonadotropins is a fundamental step in the IVF process resulting in the production of multiple follicles, with each secreting estrogen into the circulation, resulting in supraphysiological estrogen levels. There is now a growing body of evidence to support the association of elevated peak E2 levels with not only decreased success of IVF but also with increased risk of adverse perinatal outcomes including small for gestational age babies and preeclampsia (15–17). Preliminary data suggest that cryopreservation with subsequent embryo transfer in unstimulated cycles will decrease the risk of these perinatal complications (18). As reproductive medicine specialists it is mandatory that at the first consultation with the patient, a detailed full medical history including obstetric details such as, previous pregnancy complications and mode of delivery is taken. This growing body of evidence regarding supraphysiological estrogen levels in ART and subsequent pregnancy complications may in time become a factor when deciding on fresh or frozen embryo transfers for patients. Reproductive medicine specialists must aim for healthy, full term pregnancies with safe outcomes for both mother and baby. This responsibility does not end with a positive pregnancy test.

Certainly elective embryo cryopreservation and subsequent frozen embryo transfer appears to be a reasonable option for patients with high estrogen levels or early elevated progesterone levels during stimulation and particularly for those patients at high risk of ovarian hyperstimulation syndrome (OHSS) (8). It is well established that an elective "freeze-all" approach is the preferable and safe treatment option for patients at risk of OHSS.

Patients demonstrating early elevations of progesterone during superovulation may also benefit from an elective "freeze-all" approach due to the fact that progesterone is crucial to endometrial receptivity and early elevation of progesterone levels during stimulation may adversely affect embryo implantation due to changes in endometrial receptivity and gene expression (8). Studies have confirmed that late follicular phase progesterone elevation prior to hCG administration is associated with decreased pregnancy rates in IVF due to a shift in the window of implantation (19, 20). In this clinical scenario an elective "freeze-all" approach should be discussed and recommended to the patient.

During stimulation clinicians should be vigilant for risk factors of ovarian hyperstimulation syndrome and monitor serum progesterone levels closely and recommend elective "freeze-all" where appropriate. Recurrent implantation failure despite the transfer of good-quality embryos is very distressing for patients and very frustrating for clinicians. In view of the available evidence concerning endometrial receptivity and IVF/ICSI it is a sensible approach to offer these patients elective cryopreservation of their embryos with later transfer into a more physiologically normal uterine environment.

The most common treatment protocols for frozen embryo transfers include natural cycles with or without HCG trigger or endometrial preparation with hormonal treatment (artificial cycles), with or without gonadotrophin – releasing hormone agonist suppression. Recent studies comparing artificial and natural cycles concluded that the optimal means of endometrial preparation for frozen-thawed cycle remains unclear and both options may be offered to women with regular ovulatory cycles (21–24). This topic is dealt with in-depth in a further chapter.

11.3 Molecular Assessment of Endometrial Receptivity

For patients who have experienced implantation failure despite the transfer of good-quality embryos clinicians can now offer patients the endometrial receptivity assay (ERA) in the hopes of providing the patient with a "personalized" embryo transfer plan. The ERA is a technique using a customized array to identify markers of endometrial receptivity (25). It is based on the analysis of the expression of 238 genes thought to be involved in endometrial implantation (25). This test is performed in the hopes of determining a personalized "window of implantation" and is performed by obtaining an endometrial biopsy sample on day LH + 7 in a natural cycle or on the sixth day of progesterone administration during a HRT cycle. Results are expressed as prereceptive, receptive, or postreceptive. According to the result, the timing of the embryo transfer should be adjusted facilitating a "personalized" embryo transfer. The ERA test requires large randomized studies to validate its use prior to introduction into routine clinical practice.

11.4 Endometrial Cavity Fluid Identified during IVF Treatment

Endometrial cavity fluid is reported to occur during controlled ovarian stimulation in approximately 5 percent of IVF cycles (26, 27). It may be a transient finding during controlled ovarian stimulation or may be found in association with hydrosalpinx and notably, can be identified for the first time at embryo transfer. It is well established that implantation and pregnancy rates are lower if endometrial cavity fluid is associated with hydrosalpinx and if identified on the day of embryo transfer (27–29). There are many causes of fluid in the endometrial cavity including reflux from a hydrosalpinx, cervical obstruction, isthmocele/niche resulting from previous cesarean section(s), subclinical endometrial infection. However it is also important to bear in mind that it may be a physiological and transient finding. The mechanisms by which the presence of fluid within the endometrial cavity adversely affect implantation rates include embryotoxicity from endotoxins or microorganisms, reduced endometrial receptivity and not surprisingly the presence of fluid in the endometrial cavity could prove a mechanical hindrance to the apposition of the embryo to the endometrium (30). Best practice would include assessment of patients prior to commencing IVF treatment to determine if there are any risk factors which may lead to the presence of fluid in the endometrial cavity. Risk factors for tubal disease include a history of pelvic inflammatory disease, ectopic pregnancy, and endometriosis and these factors should alert clinicians to the possibility of hydrosalpinges, a well-recognized risk factor for the finding of fluid in the endometrial cavity. If the presence of fluid in the endometrial cavity proves transient with no evidence of hydrosalpinx and no fluid identified on the day of embryo transfer, it is appropriate to proceed with embryo transfer. However, if fluid is present in the endometrial cavity on the day of the planned procedure, it is best to postpone, cryopreserve the embryo and address the cause.

11.5 Embryo Transfer (ET) Procedure

The embryo transfer procedure itself is regarded as a simple procedure, but difficult transfers may occur and are associated with reduced pregnancy rates (31–33). The description of a transfer as "difficult" is subjective but is a term often used to describe transfers taking longer than usual, causing pain, requiring change of catheter, cervical dilatation, or use of a tenaculum. Many women presenting for IVF have had previous attempts at cervical instrumentation. Clinicians should ask specifically about any history of difficulty instrumenting the uterus as it may forewarn of a difficult embryo transfer. The woman may have been informed about this by previous clinicians or may remember difficult, painful, or prolonged attempts. In women with recurrent implantation failure where despite the repeated transfer of good-quality embryos, implantation does not occur, the details of previous embryo transfers should be elicited, paying particular attention to any technical difficulties encountered. In the absence of any particular difficulty encountered in previous attempts, there is no evidence that a change of embryo transfer technique will improve the implantation rate.

If the patient has a history of a difficult embryo transfer, many clinics will perform a "trial" embryo transfer procedure. This may be described as the passage of an empty embryo transfer catheter through the cervix, thus mimicking the real embryo transfer procedure (34, 35). Very useful information can be gleaned from the "trial" procedure including the type of speculum and embryo catheter best suited to the patient, need for a tenaculum, and very importantly, the direction and curve of the catheter required to negotiate the internal cervical os. This information is recorded and will assist the clinician in ensuring a smooth embryo transfer on the assigned transfer day. A randomized controlled trail (RCT) involving 335 patients demonstrated that the patients who had a trial embryo transfer procedure had a significantly lower incidence of "difficult" embryo transfer and significantly higher implantation and pregnancy rates (35). The trial procedure can be performed before commencing ovarian stimulation or immediately before the actual transfer.

In an effort to preempt potential problems on the day of embryo transfer clinicians should take into account risk factors for a difficult procedure such as cervical stenosis following cervical surgery, acute anteversion/retroversion or to acute anteflexion/retroflexion of the uterus. Clinicians should be aware of several techniques which may be employed when difficulty is encountered.

Performing embryo transfers under transabdominal ultrasound guidance has many advantages and has been shown to increase ongoing clinical pregnancy rates (36). Many ET catheters have echogenic tips facilitating direct visualization with ultrasound at the cervico-uterine angle which can facilitate insertion of the catheter. Ultrasound guidance will assist in the identification of cases where the catheter tip curls backward, when difficulty is encountered passing through the cervical os and will prevent the inadvertent injection of the embryo into the cervical canal.

Reproductive medicine specialists commonly see patients with secondary infertility with a history of having had one or more previous lower uterine segment cesarean sections and with ultrasound confirmation of an isthmocele/niche. The presence of an isthmocele/niche may render the embryo transfer procedure technically more difficult. Clinicians first need to be aware of its presence and perform the transfer under ultrasound guidance to ensure the catheter bypasses the isthmocele and enters the uterine cavity.

Transabdominal ultrasound guidance will require a second operator and the need to bladder fill. Bladder filling is a simple measure which in itself may be advantageous for those women with acute anteversion or anteflexion of the uterus but will not be helpful in cases of acute retroversion or retroflexion where an empty bladder is preferable (34).

The application of a tenaculum to the anterior lip of the cervix and applying traction gently downward may help to straighten an acutely flexed uterus but may compromise pregnancy rates by inducing uterine contractions (37).

If difficulty is encountered negotiating the internal cervical os a rigid embryo transfer catheter as opposed to a soft catheter may be more beneficial and may assist in avoiding the need to apply a tenaculum to the cervix (38). If the transfer procedure still proves difficult despite employing the above described measures it is best to abandon the procedure, (re) freeze the embryo and formulate a management plan. Alternative methods to transcervical embryo transfer include transmyometrial and tubal transfer but should be reserved for cases which are extremely difficult or impossible (39–41).

11.6 Conclusion

Embryo transfer is regarded generally as a routine, simple procedure but yet many clinicians experience difficulty on the assigned day of embryo transfer. Management of these cases is critical to the success of the procedure. When planning the transfer the findings during the stimulation cycle must be considered and the couples prior treatment history has to be reviewed in order to offer them the best advice as to a fresh embryo transfer or to proceed with an elective "freeze-all." In planning an embryo transfer, as in all aspects of medicine we must individualize patient care as "one size does not fit all."

References

1. Roque M, Lattes K, Serra S, et al. Fresh embryo transfer versus frozen embryo transfer in in vitro fertilization cycles: a systematic review and meta-analysis. Fertil Steril 2013;99(1):156–162.

2. Roque M, Valle M, Guimaraes F, et al. Freeze-all policy: fresh vs. frozen-thawed embryo transfer. Fertil Steril 2015:103 (5):1190–1193.

3. Bourgain C, Devroey P. The endometrium in stimulated cycles for IVF. Hum Reprod Update 2003;9:515–522.

4. Devroey P, Bourgain C, Macklon NS, et al. Reproductive biology and IVF: ovarian stimulation and endometrial receptivity. Trends Endocrinol Metab 2004;15:84–90.

5. Kolibianakis E, Bourgain C, Albano C, et al. Effect of ovarian stimulation with recombinant follicle-stimulating hormone, gonadotropin release hormone antagonists, and human chorionic gonadotropin on endometrial maturation on the day of oocyte pick-up. Fertil Steril 2002;78:1025–1029.

6. Nikas G, Develioglu OH, Toner JP, et al. Endometrial pinopodes indicate a shift in

the window of receptivity in IVF cycles. Hum Reprod 1999;14:787–792.

7. Simon C, Velasco JJG, Valbuena D, et al. Increasing uterine receptivity by decreasing estradiol levels during the pre-implantation period in high responders with the use of a follicle stimulating hormone step down regimen. Fertil Steril 1998;70:234–239.

8. Weinerman R, Mainigi M. Why we should transfer frozen instead of fresh embryos: the translational rationale. Fertil Steril 2014;102(1):10–18.

9. Liu Y, Lee KF, Ng EH, et al. Gene expression profiling of human peri-implantation endometria between natural and stimulated cycles. Fertil Steril 2008;90:2152–2164.

10. Haouzi D, Assou S, Mahmoud K, et al. Gene expression profile of human endometrial receptivity: comparison between natural and stimulated cycles for the same patients. *Hum Reprod* 2009;24:1436–1445.

11. Maheshwari A, Bhattacharya S. Elective frozen replacement cycles for all: ready for prime time? Hum Reprod 2013;28(1):6–9.

12. Shapiro BS, Daneshmand ST, Garner FC, et al. Freezes-all can be a superior therapy to another fresh cycle in patients with prior fresh blastocyst implantation failure. Reprod Biomed Online 2014;29:286–290.

13. Roque M, Valle M, Guimaraes F, et al. Freeze-all policy: fresh vs. frozen-thawed embryo transfer. Fertil Steril 2015;103:1190–1193.

14. Magdi Y, Damen A, Fathi A, et al. Revisiting the management of recurrent implantation failure through freeze-all policy. Fertil Steril 2017;108(1):72–77.

15. Farhi J, Ben-Haroush A, Andrawus N, et al. High serum oestradiol concentrations in IVF cycles increase the risk of pregnancy complications related to abnormal placentation. Reprod Biomed Online 2010;21:331–337.

16. Joo BS, Park SH, An BM, et al. Serum estradiol levels during controlled ovarian hyperstimulation influence the pregnancy outcome of in vitro fertilization in a concentration-dependent manner. Fertil Steril 2010;93:442–446.

17. Imudia AN, Awonuga AO, Doyle JO, et al. Peak serum estradiol level during controlled ovarian hyperstimulation is associated with increased risk of small for gestational age and preeclampsia in singleton pregnancies after in vitro fertilization. Fertil Steril 2012;97:1374–1379.

18. Imudia AN, Awonuga AO, Kaimal AJ, et al. Elective cryopreservation of all embryos with subsequent cryothaw embryo transfer in patients at risk for ovarian hyperstimulation syndrome reduces the risk of adverse obstetric outcomes: a preliminary study. Fertil Steril 2013;99:168–173.

19. Bosch E, Labarta E, Crespo J, et al. Circulating progesterone levels and ongoing pregnancy rates in controlled ovarian stimulation cycles for in vitro fertilization: analysis of over 4000 cycles. Hum Reprod 2010;25:2092–2100.

20. Al-Azemi M, Kyrou D, Kolibianakis EM, et al. Elevated progesterone during ovarian stimulation for IVF. Reprod Biomed Online 2012;24:381–388.

21. Ghobara T, Gelbaya TA, Ayeleke RO. Cycle regimens for frozen-thawed embryo transfer. Cochrane Database Syst Rev 2017;5(7):CD003414.

22. Groenewoud E, Cantineau A, Kollen BJ, et al. What is the optimal means of preparing the endometrium in frozen-thawed embryo transfer cycles? A systematic review and meta-analysis. Hum Reprod Update 2013;19(5):458–470.

23. Groenewoud E, Cohlen B, Macklon N. Programming the endometrium for deferred transfer of cryopreserved embryos: hormone replacement versus modified natural cycles. Fertil Steril 2018;109(5):768–774.

24. Groenewoud E, Cohlen B, Al-Oraiby A, et al. A randomized controlled, non-inferiority trial of modified natural versus artificial cycle for cryo-thawed

embryo transfer. Hum Reprod 2016;31 (7):1483–1492.

25. Casper R, Haas J, Hsieh TB, et al. Recent advances in in vitro fertilization. F1000Res 2017;6:1616.

26. Lee RK, Yu Sl, Chih YF, et al. Effect of endometrial cavity fluid on clinical pregnancy rate in tubal embryo transfer (TET). J Assist Reprod Genet 2006;23:229–234.

27. Chien LW, Au HK, Xiao J, et al. Fluid accumulation within the uterine cavity reduces pregnancy rates in women undergoing IVF. Hum Reprod 2012;17:351–356.

28. Levi AJ, Segars JH, Miller BT, et al. Endometrial cavity fluid is associated with poor ovarian response and increased cancellation rates in ART cycles. Hum Reprod 2001;16:2610–2615.

29. Akman MA, Erden HF, Bahceci M. Endometrial fluid visualized through ultrasonography during ovarian stimulation in IVF cycles impairs the outcome in tubal factor, but not PCOH, patients. Hum Reprod 2005;20:906–909.

30. Coomarasamy A. Endometrial cavity fluid identified during IVF treatment. In: *Assisted Reproduction Techniques: Challenges and Management Options.* Ed. Sharif K, Coomarasamy A. Blackwell, 2012:249–251.

31. Mains L, Van Voorhis BJ. Optimizing the technique of embryo transfer. Fertil Steril 2010;94:785–790.

32. Sallam HN, Agameya AF, Rahman AF, et al. Impact of technical difficulties, choice of catheter, and the presence of blood on the success of embryo transfer–experience from a single provider. J Assist Reprod Genet 2003;20:135–142.

33. Tomas C, Tikkinen K, Tuomivaara L, et al. The degree of difficulty of embryo transfer is an independent factor for predicting pregnancy. Hum Reprod 2002;17:2632–2635.

34. Sharif K, Afnan M, Lenton W. Mock embryo transfer with a full bladder immediately before the real transfer for in-vitro fertilization treatment: the Birmingham experience of 113 cases. Hum Reprod 1995;10:1715–1718.

35. Mansour R, Aboulghar M, Serour G. Dummy embryo transfer: a technique that minimizes the problems of embryo transfer and improves the pregnancy rate in human in vitro fertilization. Fertil Steril 1990;54:678–681.

36. Brown JA, Buckingham K, About-Setta A, et al. Ultrasound versus "clinical touch" for catheter guidance during embryo transfer in women. Cochrane Database Syst Rev 2010;1:CD006107.

37. Lesny P, Killick SR, Robinson J, et al. Junctional zone contractions and embryo transfer: is it safe to use a tenaculum? Hum Reprod 1999;14:2367–2370.

38. Abou-Setta AM, Al-Inany HG, Mansour RT, et al. Soft versus firm embryo transfer catheters for assisted reproduction: a systematic review and meta-analysis. Hum Reprod 2005;20:3114–3121.

39. Sharif K, Afnan M, Lenton W, et al. Transmyometrial embryo transfer after difficult immediate mock transcervical transfer. Fertil Steril 1996;65:1071–1074.

40. Yang YS, Melinda S, Ho HN, et al. Effect of the number and depth of embryos transferred and unilateral or bilateral transfer in tubal embryo transfer (TET). J Assist Reprod Genet 1992;9:534–538.

41. Sharif K. Difficult embryo transfer. In: *Assisted Reproduction Techniques: Challenges and Management Options.* Ed. Sharif K, Coomarasamy A. Blackwell, 2012:252–256.

Index